The Art of Surfing

A Training Manual for the Developing and Competitive Surfer

Help Us Keep This Guide Up to Date

Every effort has been made by the author and editors to make this guide as accurate and useful as possible. However, many things can change after a guide is published—regulations change, techniques evolve, organizations come under new management, and so on.

We would love to hear from you concerning your experiences with this guide and how you feel it could be improved and kept up to date. While we may not be able to respond to all comments and suggestions, we'll take them to heart and we'll also make certain to share them with the author. Please send your comments and suggestions to the following address:

The Globe Pequot Press
Reader Response/Editorial Department
P.O. Box 480
Guilford, CT 06437

Or you may e-mail us at:

editorial@globe-pequot.com

Thanks for your input.

The Art of Surfing

A Training Manual for the Developing and Competitive Surfer

RAUL GUISADO

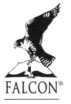

FALCON®

GUILFORD, CONNECTICUT
HELENA, MONTANA

AN IMPRINT OF THE GLOBE PEQUOT PRESS

All interior photos courtesy of author Raul Guisado.
Illustrations by Kendra Joseph
Text design by Casey Shain
Images on pages xii, 66, and 68–69, and spot images
   © 2002–2003 www.clipart.com.

Library of Congress Cataloging-in-Publication Data is available.
ISBN 0-7627-2466-8

Manufactured in the United States of America
First Edition/Third Printing

This book is dedicated to Aaron Martin,
for showing us all how to live each day to the fullest.

CONTENTS

ACKNOWLEDGMENTS

I'd like to thank the following people for their time, energy, advice, and support:

Toby Corey and family, Raul Guisado Sr., Vin Gulisano, Wendell Jones, Kendra Joseph, Jeff Klaas, Kristina Koznick, Jeremy Marshall, John Mulligan, Josh Oshinsky, Matt Partain, Evelyn Rehklau, John Rehklau, Dan Stripp, Daren Wein, and Donna Wueste.

A special thanks to Ross Cuyler and his staff at Fiberglass Santa Cruz.

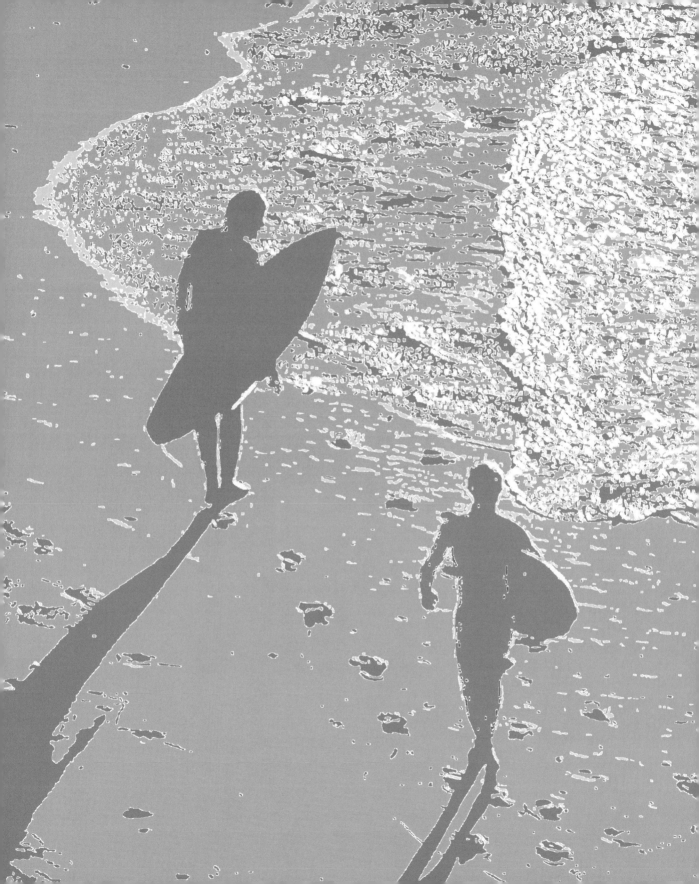

INTRODUCTION

Whether you're a pro surfer who wants to win a world title, a competitive surfer who wants to turn pro, or a recreational surfer who just wants to shred over your friends, the information in this book will help you reach your goals!

Surfing has evolved from its status not long ago as a relatively obscure pastime to one of the fastest-growing sports in the world. Today there are several million surfers across the globe. Despite this growing popularity, however, the sport has yet to gain the respect it deserves in the athletic community. In fact, surfing is a skill sport that's not only a tremendous amount of fun, but also demanding both physically and psychologically.

My goal in writing this book is to add, in some small way, to the body of knowledge of this incredible sport. I hope to expose surfers to training principles that have proven effective in a variety of other sports. Surfing will continue to evolve rapidly and will require an open mind in the years to come. Competitive surfing will only become more and more competitive as more marketing dollars are dedicated to the sport and more is at stake in each contest. Increases in funding and attention will draw more and better athletes to the sport, and surfers will have to train harder and smarter in the future.

What's clear is that this is a cutting-edge sport, and it's about time that surfers have access to and use the same coaching principles already employed in more established and traditional sports. For years, the majority of surfers have done very little out of the water to improve their performance. In contrast, athletes in other skill sports have for decades been utilizing state-of-the art sports science to refine technique and fitness. Competitive and recreational surfers who want to improve can benefit from a variety of relatively simple and easy-to-implement performance enhancement methods. If all we do is surf, we're unable to challenge ourselves beyond the demands of our surfing. Moreover, without this added challenge we're less likely to make rapid or significant improvements in our performance.

As in other sports, few athletes in the sport of surfing are able to rely on talent alone; ultimately only those who train intelligently will succeed. Surfers must continually strive to take their skills to the next

> What's clear is that this is a cutting-edge sport, and it's about time that surfers have access to and use the same coaching principles already employed in more established and traditional sports.

level. If we do, the overall skill level of the sport will never plateau. In order to keep up with the development of the sport, you must identify your strengths and weaknesses as an athlete and look for ways to improve. Once you understand what you need to work on, you can develop strategies for becoming a more complete surfer.

Progress in any endeavor is an ongoing process, and those at the pinnacle of any activity are proactive rather than reactive. In other words, reaching your potential requires taking the initiative to continually seek out and implement knowledge that will help you reach your goals. Become a student of the sport and you'll soon find that surfing at a high level is dependent on a number of interrelated factors. For example, great surfers possess a tremendous amount of wave and ocean knowledge, which aids them in wave selection. They know how their equipment and diet affects their surfing. Most advanced surfers are able to analyze the body positions, style, and technique of others, and take time to watch video of their own surfing as well. They're aerobically and anaerobically fit in order to meet the cardiovascular demands of the sport. They're also flexible, stable, agile, strong, powerful, and mentally prepared to adapt to ever-changing wave shapes, perform complex maneuvers, and overcome unforeseen physical and psychological challenges. Above all, a majority of accomplished surfers are students of the sport and are proactive. They lead rather than follow and are rarely content with their present level of surfing.

The Art of Surfing will give you ideas for ways you can take your surfing to the next level. If you're serious about improving, this book can

be a great resource—a textbook, if you will—in your development as a surfer. The first chapter is dedicated to the basics of surfing in the hope of filling any gaps in nitty-gritty knowledge and getting everyone on the "same page," so to speak. Whether you've been surfing all your life or have only recently gotten hooked, I urge you to pay close attention to the information in that chapter. Even though a great deal of it may sound familiar, it will help lay the groundwork for this book's performance enhancement sections. The remainder of the book was written with the intermediate to advanced surfer in mind. I aim to empower both the recreational and competitive athlete and, as a result, improve the way surfers prepare to reach their goals. Knowledge of performance enhancement techniques can help you surf better every day without injury, get you ready for a two-week surf trip, or aid you in reaching competitive aspirations.

My hope is that this book will not only make you a better surfer but also increase your enjoyment of the sport. As you probably already know, surfing can be a truly transforming experience: There are few sports that inspire and evoke as strong a connection with our planet as does this one. Whatever your motivation in reading this book, I hope you find it useful. May the joy of riding waves keep your soul smiling for eternity!

Chapter 1

THE BASICS Surfing Fundamentals

Surfing generates in its participants an almost religious awe for the beauty and energy of waves, and of the sea that gives birth to these mysterious forces of nature. —*Paul Holmes, longtime surfer*

The goal of this chapter is to cover the essentials or "nuts and bolts" of surfing. We'll discuss the history of surfing, ocean knowledge, equipment, etiquette and the fundamentals of riding waves. It's information that many surfers acquire within their first few years in the sport, through experience and from veteran surfers. The objective is to make sure we're all "on the same page," so we can discuss ways to take your surfing to the next level!

A BRIEF HISTORY OF SURFING

In order to understand the sport of surfing, it's important to first learn a little bit about its history.

Sometime before 1500 A.D. kings, queens, men, and women of the Sandwich Isles enjoyed *he'enalu,* wave sliding. The boards were made of solid wood, up to 18 feet long, and could weigh as much as 150 pounds. In 1778, Captain Cook reported finding the natives of the Hawaiian Islands surfing. Unfortunately, white settlers of Hawaii considered surfing heathen, and the sport was nearly extinct by the end of the 1800s.

The Waikiki area of Oahu was the center of surfing for the few who still enjoyed the sport.

Then, in the early 1900s a surfing revival began. In 1907 George Freeth, of Hawaiian and Irish heritage, moved from Waikiki to Redondo Beach, California. He surfed as a publicity stunt to promote the opening of the Redondo–LA railroad. Freeth stayed in California to become the first lifeguard and is credited with teaching the first Californians to ride waves. In the same year, Alexander Hume Ford formed the mainly Caucasian Outrigger Canoe Club in Waikiki "for the purpose of preserving surfing on boards and in Hawaiian canoes." In 1911, Hui Nalu Surfing Club was officially organized in Waikiki to promote the sport of surfing among Hawaiians. Shortly thereafter, in 1915, Duke Kahanamoku gave a surfing exhibition while in Australia for a swimming competition. He also impressed spectators in California, New York, and New Jersey and can be credited for sparking what would eventually become international awareness of the sport. Duke went on to make movies in Hollywood and is considered the father of the modern surfing era.

Surfing started to become very popular in Southern California in the 1920s. Many credit the advent of the lighter boards produced by people like Tom Blake. In 1935, Blake put a small fin on the rear of a surfboard, making it much more maneuverable. The design evolution continued when in 1946 Preston "Pete" Peterson built a fiberglass-and-foam surfboard. And in 1949, Bob Simmons built the first foam-and-fiberglass boards to be commercially successful. His boards became the prototype for the models to follow.

The 1950s are known as the Golden Age of Modern Surfing. Board manufacturing became completely commercialized, and surfing transformed from a pastime to a multimillion-dollar industry. Perhaps one of the most significant developments of that decade came in 1952 when Jack O'Neill sold the first wet suit in Northern California. Up to that point surfing in places like Santa Cruz in the winter months, when the surf is the best, was limited to a small crew of truly committed and perpetually cold individuals. Wet suits made the sport much more inviting and have since prolonged the average surf session in cold-water parts of the world considerably. In 1953, Southern Californians Dave Velzy and Hap Jacobs began making the only commercially available balsa wood boards. These boards became very popular for being lightweight, aesthetically pleasing, and durable. Balsa wood, however, would eventually play a much smaller role in surfboard manufacture as a result of Hobie Alter's and Gordon Clark's creation of the first foam surfboard blanks in 1958. These blanks were easily shaped, required only one to three thin strips of balsa wood running down the center, and accelerated surfboard design into the 1960s.

In that decade, surf movies flourished and surfing grew even more popular, with California considered the capital. Boards were being made ever smaller and lighter. Since the 1970s, there have been numerous innovations in equipment, style, and contests. Surfing has become an estab-

lished sport, with surfers, shapers, and contests found all over the globe. A sport that originated and was enjoyed more than 500 years ago by Polynesian royalty is now keeping millions smiling and young at heart.

THE BREAK

One thing all great surfers have in common is their awareness that waves are incredible forces of nature. The ocean can be immensely beautiful, inspirational, fascinating, and powerful all at the same time. One of the most alluring aspects of surfing is the electrifying feeling of being at one with a wave and adapting to its ever-changing contours. To achieve this oneness, be safe, and excel in the sport, however, you must exercise a great deal of respect for the ocean. What follows is meant to help us better understand the nature of the dynamic, watery terrain we as surfers depend on.

The key to enjoying surfing safely and successfully for years to come is to become a true *waterman* or *waterwoman*—an extremely proficient ocean swimmer and surfer. The first step in your development as a waterperson is to become a student of the ocean and waves. Surfing is an enormous amount of fun, but keep in mind that you're ultimately playing by the ocean's rules. Knowledge helps eliminate surprises and will result in higher-quality surf sessions.

Ocean Safety

Surfing is an incredibly fun sport that can be enjoyed by people of all ages. Because you're dealing with the sometimes unpredictable force of ocean waves, however, it's important to think safety first.

The Golden Rule in Ocean Safety: *Mai huli 'oe I kokua o ke kai!*—Hawaiian for "Never turn your back on the ocean!"

Before we go any farther, I want to emphasize the importance of being knowledgeable about your surroundings while surfing. At the same time, I don't intend to paint a picture of surfing as an overly hazardous or "extreme" sport. Any activity can be extreme if you're in over your head. In fact, one of the goals of this book is to expand your ability so that what you once considered extreme is now within your comfort zone.

There are days when the waves are small and mellow, and all seems harmless and calm. There are also days when the ocean can be a volatile and even destructive force. It's important to set aside machismo and ego at times and realize that ultimately the ocean will always win. Wave action, at any worthwhile surf spot, can at times humble the most experienced waterperson. One of the differences between waterpeople and *kooks* (inexperienced or disrespectful surfers) is that waterpeople can make informed decisions and predetermine the level of risk they will face. Certain breaks and conditions are suited for particular levels of surfers. It's similar to the way that ski areas designate their runs for differing levels of skiers and snowboarders. There are some days when no one should venture into the water. The

The Surfrider Foundation

The Surfrider Foundation is a non-profit organization dedicated to protecting our oceans. Its national office is in San Clemente, California, but the foundation has active chapters all over the world.

Local chapters act to protect the coast in their community. For example, they take ocean water samples to determine bacteria levels and publish the results of their water testing in local newspapers and on the Web. They welcome volunteers who love oceans, waves, and beaches. Surfrider chapter locations include:

- East Coast: numerous chapters from Florida to New England
- Great Lakes
- Gulf Coast
- Islands of Oahu, Maui, and Puerto Rico
- West Coast: numerous chapters from San Diego to Seattle
- Australia
- Brazil
- France
- Japan

For more information, visit their Web site at www.surfrider.org.

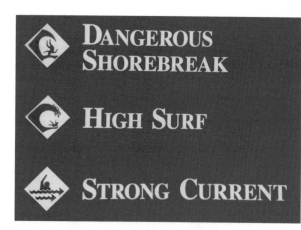

Sign showing dangerous water conditions.

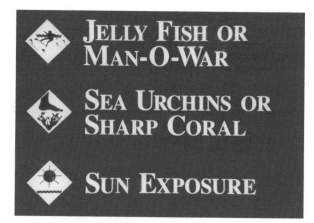

Sign showing other beach hazards.

experienced surfer's most valuable tool regarding ocean safety is common sense and sound judgment. If in doubt, just stay out!

When you're first learning how to surf, it's advisable to stick to beaches with lifeguards. They can be a wealth of information for you, as well as increasing the safety level of the sport enormously. Check with lifeguards regarding conditions, and definitely observe all posted warning signs. Many lifeguards will tell you that it's essential to watch the surf for at least fifteen minutes before entering the water. And unless you're an experienced waterperson and a strong swimmer, you should never swim, bodysurf, bodyboard, sailboard, or surf in waves more than waist high.

Buddy System

Another way to make the sport safer is to avoid surfing alone. As with sports such as scuba diving, kayaking, snorkeling, skiing, snowboarding, and rock climbing, surfers at every level should try to employ the "buddy system" by surfing with a friend. You and your buddy can keep an eye on each other and offer assistance in the

event that something unforeseeable happens. Another benefit is that you can improve from surfing with someone who's better than you. Of course, the best reason to surf with a friend is the most obvious. You can laugh with (or at) each other, and on a good day share your stoke!

First-Aid Tips

There are a few simple first-aid tips everyone who ventures into the ocean should know.

The most common injuries incurred by surfers are:

- *Surfboard bruises and cuts.* Surfboards can quickly turn into projectiles when they fly into the air or are pushed by a wall of water. To protect yourself and others, *always* be in control of your board. When you fall, it's a good idea to protect your head with your hands and arms. Beginners should use foam boards opposed to fiberglass. Shortboarders should apply protectors to their fins as well as to the nose of the board to avoid being stabbed in a fall. Swelling from bruises can be treated by applying ice to the area. Cuts should be cleaned, disinfected, and covered immediately.

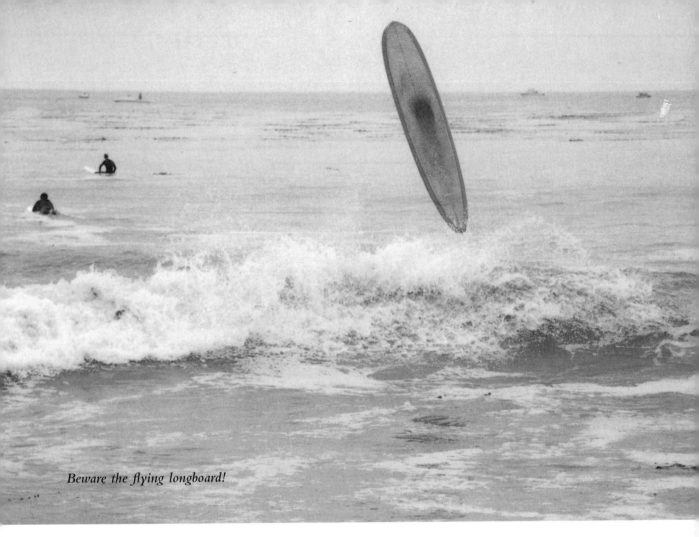

Beware the flying longboard!

- *Rock bruises, scrapes, and cuts.* Rocks in shallow water or on the shore have left a dent in many a surfboard and surfer. Most commonly, injury occurs while trying to enter and exit the water. A lot of shoreline rocks are covered by moss and become extremely slippery when wet. It's advisable to find a safe—preferably sandy—area to enter and exit the water, especially at high tide.
- *Coral scrapes and cuts.* The biggest problem when coming into contact with coral is the risk of infection. Bacteria from the seawater enter the wound and begin to grow. Signs of local infection include pain, redness, warmth, and pus. Wash cuts with fresh water and soap within the first hour of injury to prevent infection. Also, apply antibiotic ointment and cover the area until the cut begins to heal.
- *Sea urchin spikes.* The most common sea urchin encounters occur when walking near the shore. Large urchin spikes are the size of a pencil lead and need to be removed by a physician. The small spikes are the size of a sewing needle and cannot be removed. The good news is that the body readily dissolves the small spikes in a couple of weeks. A toxin released by the urchin upon contact causes the pain. To destroy the toxin and relieve pain, soak the injured area in hot water or vinegar for fifteen minutes a few times a day.
- *Jellyfish or Portuguese man-of-war stings.* These guys can hurt! The worst part is that they're

difficult to see and can suddenly surprise you with a sting. Avoid rubbing the affected area; this will only make matters worse. Instead, wash the skin off gently with alcohol to prevent further stinging. The most effective way to destroy the toxin is to apply meat tenderizer paste for fifteen minutes. If you develop large areas of hives or experience difficulty in breathing, seek medical attention immediately.

Wave Formation

The most common reason why waves form is wind in the open ocean. Waves breaking against a shore are called *surf*. The surf we enjoy is the end of a journey of energy that may have originated thousands of miles away. Waves are formed as variations in air pressure force gusty winds down upon the water's surface. If the wind is strong and steady enough, it will form chop over a large area. This chop is referred to as a *sea*. As the sea is blown downwind, the waves become longer, smoother, and more organized, taking the form of what we call a *swell*. A swell is what we recognize as the marching *lines* of energy that travel across the open ocean. An incoming swell usually means better surf. When this wave energy hits shallow water, it begins to crest and form a breaking wave. This is when all the wave's energy finally moves a significant amount of water. In other words, from the swell's origination point until the wave breaks, energy has been moving through the ocean without actually displacing the water. It's the energy that has traveled hundreds or thousands of miles since the creation of the swell, not the actual water molecules. Waves generated by the wind may range in height from less than an inch to as much as 60 feet

Earthquakes and volcanic eruptions beneath the ocean cause other waves. Waves formed by underwater earthquakes are known as seismic sea waves or (in Japanese) *tsunamis*. Near the coast, tsunamis may become very large and cause a lot of damage, but in the deep open ocean the eye cannot detect them. In extreme cases, tsunamis can be as high as 100 feet and travel up to 600 miles per hour. Fortunately, these "great waves" are quite rare, and scientists have become pretty good at forecasting them.

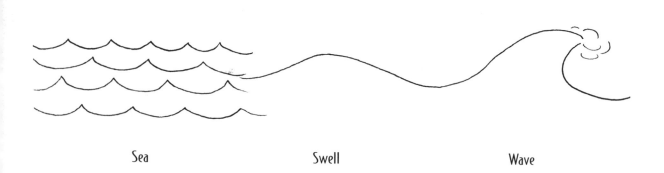

Sea   Swell   Wave

Progression from a sea, to a swell, to a wave.

The lines of a swell.

Anatomy of a Wave

Throughout the years, surfers have named the different parts of a wave.

The highest part of a wave is called the *crest* or *peak*. The lowest part is called the *trough* or *pit*. The front of the wave is called the *face,* and the back of the wave is generally referred to as simply the back.

The *curl* is the part of the wave that is breaking. *Lip* is a term used to describe the very tip of a cresting wave that curls or plunges down. *Wall* is a general term used to refer to the area of the face that has yet to break. A *section* is a portion or an area of a wave. The *pocket* is the section of the wall just ahead of the curl. It's usually the steepest part of the wave and the most desirable place to surf. If you can stay in or near the pocket, you can generate maximal speed and enjoy a longer ride. The *shoulder* or *flats* is the less steep section of the wave face away from the breaking part.

Wave Measurement

In the sport of surfing, wave measurement varies considerably. Some folks measure waves from the face of the wave, while others, especially in Hawaii, measure from the back. Essentially, all wave measurement by a surfer is a "guesstimate." It mostly becomes an issue in storytelling, contests, and photo shoots.

Why all this variation? It's because waves are dynamic and change in width, height, and shape as they approach shore. To complicate things further, wave size differs depending on the angle of the observer. I've heard it said that perhaps the

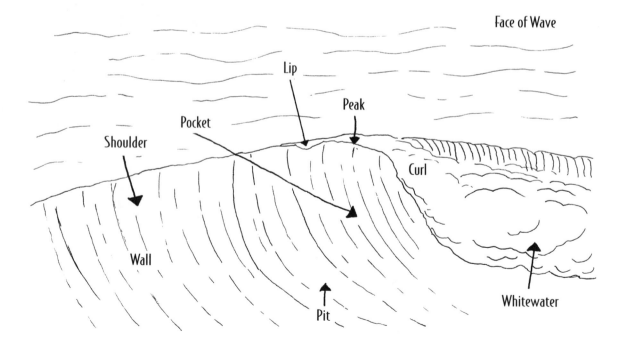

The anatomy of a wave.

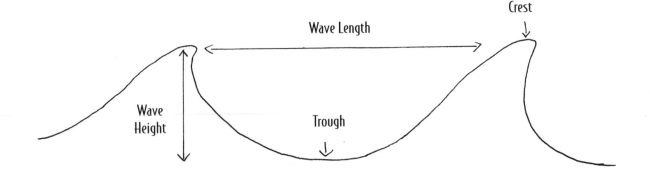

Wave measurement.

units of wave measurement should be fear rather than feet.

Regardless of your choice of measurement technique while in the water, it's important to understand how it's done in surf predictions. Satellites, ocean buoys, vessel reports, and meteorological data have become fairly accurate at predicting surf. These surf reports usually describe what direction the swell is traveling, the time interval between waves, and the wave height. *Wave height* is determined by measuring the vertical distance between the crest and trough. *Wave length* is the distance between two successive wave crests. Swell data will be most useful to those who know the spot they're surfing and have experience determining wave shape.

Wave Shape

Wave shape can vary drastically from day to day at the same spot. Swell size, speed, and direction; tides; currents; the curve and shape of the shore; kelp; and wind conditions all affect shape. Every surf spot has a unique set of variables with which you need to become familiar.

Areas with long, gradual rises from deep to

shallow water usually result in what is known as a *peeling* wave. A peeling wave breaks easily down the face or frontside of the wave, spilling or toppling over. It appears to crumble or peel along its length and is excellent for learning how to surf.

Breaks with a more abrupt change from deep to shallow water usually result in what is known as a *tubing* wave. A tubing wave breaks from top to bottom as the swell peaks more quickly and pitches the crest down the wave face. This type of wave creates the hollow *tube* or *barrel* section that an advanced surfer enters. Getting *barreled* is one of the ultimate experiences in surfing. The term *hollow* is used to describe this concave and steep wave face shape. The term *sucky* is also used to describe wave conditions that are hollow and breaking in shallow water. *Gnarly* is a slang term used to describe large, heavy, thick-lipped or difficult waves.

When waves break all at once along their entire face, they are referred to as being *closed out*. Such waves are not ideal for surfing—you end up merely riding the *whitewater* or broken part of a wave that has already peaked and toppled over. Sometimes catching the whitewater can work to your advantage if it's a wave that will break twice. Such waves are called *reforms* because they have already broken, but—depending on how much energy they have and the shape of the bottom—they can reform to break again.

Tides

Being familiar with the spot you will surf and how different tides affect it is essential to experiencing quality surf sessions.

Tides are related to the moon's cycles and occur in any large body of water, but they're most prominent along the coast. In most places, the tide rises and falls twice a day. The maximum and minimum levels of rise and fall are called high and low tide, respectively. It takes roughly six hours for rising water to reach high tide and approximately another six or so to reach low tide again. This sequence is called the tidal cycle and is repeated every twelve hours and twenty-five minutes. The amount of change in the water level during the cycle is known as the tidal range. During the first and last quarter of the moon's cycle, called a neap tide, there is minimal difference between high and low tides. When there's a full- or new-moon cycle, known as a spring tide, there's a bigger difference between high and low tides.

Most surf shops can provide you with a book that lists the times high and low tide will occur each day for the entire year in their local area. This can help you plan your surfing session, because changes in water depth at the points where waves break can significantly alter the shape of the wave. For example, if the tide is too high and a significant swell isn't on the way, the waves are likely to be small and have little power. On the other hand, when the tide is too low

there may not be enough water for decent waves to form. In areas that experience a considerable amount of kelp growth, a very low tide can also result in a great deal of the green stuff at the surface. This can make surfing a real challenge: When struck by a surfboard's fin, kelp acts like a speed bump.

The more experience you have surfing a particular break, and the more you know current swell data and wind conditions, the better you'll be able to predict what tide height will make for the optimal surf session!

Currents

If you've spent any time in or around the ocean you're probably already familiar with the concept of ocean currents. Forces such as the wind, wave action, and changes in tides, result in water movement or currents. Unlike swell energy that travels through the water, currents can sweep objects both on the bottom and at the surface in the direction the water is flowing. For example, currents are what cause boats to drift and sand bars to shift.

Currents can vary significantly in terms of strength and direction. Therefore, everyone who ventures into the ocean needs to be aware of currents to prevent being swept out to sea or into an area where waves are breaking onto rocks or into cliffs. Scuba divers, for instance, might start their dives by swimming against the current so they can expend less energy on their return. A strong current that moves parallel to shore can affect us when we're surfing because it can make it difficult for us to hold our position while we wait for waves.

After waves have broken on shore the water needs a way to flow back out to sea. The path of least resistance for the water to return is the low-

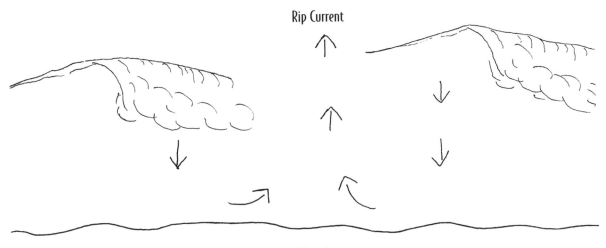

A rip current.

est spot in the shore. This movement of water can form what's referred to as a *rip current*. Rip currents can be very strong and are important for ocean goers to identify. Each year, many swimmers and surfers are swept out to sea by rip currents because they become fatigued trying to swim against the flow. The key is to swim across the rip current or parallel to shore until you've broken free from its pull.

Wind Conditions

What direction the wind is blowing can greatly affect wave shape.

In the morning or evening, there tends to be little or no wind, and the surf is more likely to be *glassy*. This term refers to the incredibly smooth appearance of incoming swells and waves—ideal conditions for surfing.

An *onshore* wind is one that blows from the ocean and is usually the least favorable direction. Strong onshore winds often result in *blown-out*

surf: waves that have been made bumpy or flattened by the wind. This type of surf is also referred to as *mush*.

A *sideshore* wind blows across the swell, and although it's better than an onshore wind, it can also lead to deteriorating conditions.

An *offshore* wind blows from the shore into the surf and can enhance wave shape. An offshore wind helps hold up the incoming waves, giving them cleaner, more ridable faces.

Types of Breaks

Surf spots—areas where surfable waves form— are also called *breaks*. Wave energy will break differently depending on the tide, the swell direction, and, just as importantly, the characteristics of the shore bottom.

- *Beach breaks* are areas where waves are breaking very close to shore. Often such breaks are very steep and hollow, making them difficult to surf. Beach breaks are often frequented by bodysurfers, bodyboarders, skimboarders, and, depending on the quality of the wave, short-boarders.

- *Sand breaks* are areas where waves break over a sandbar. These breaks can be altered, because sand shifts and can look very different from time to time. Sand breaks are usually found closer to shore and create smaller waves.
- *Reef breaks* are areas where waves break over a coral or rocky reef. Coral reef breaks tend to occur in shallow water and can create some of the most spectacular barrels in the world. The majority of the famous island breaks in the world are coral reef breaks.
- *Point breaks* are areas where waves break at a part of the shore that extends outward. These breaks tend to be larger and more consistent than other breaks because they are the first areas of shallow water that a swell hits. Often a swell will wrap around a point, providing more than one surfable peak.
- *Inside breaks* are areas where waves break relatively close to shore. Because they don't require very much energy to paddle to, these breaks tend to be the most popular for surfing. However, because they are closer to shore, inside breaks near rock outcroppings or cliffs may not be safe for novice surfers when the tide is high.
- *Outside breaks* are areas of somewhat shallow water where waves break farther from shore. These breaks can create some of the largest and most powerful waves. Because the water is deeper than inside breaks, outside breaks usually require a deeper groundswell in order for waves to form.
- *Lefts* are waves that break from the peak to the surfer's left. This usually means you'll get a more desirable and longer ride by turning left

after catching the wave. The quality of a left at any surf spot is dependent on the swell size and direction as well as the tide, current, and wind conditions.
- *Rights,* as you may guess, are waves that break from the peak to the surfer's right. This usually means you'll get a more desirable and longer ride by turning right after catching the wave. The quality of a right at any surf spot is dependent on the swell size and direction as well as the tide, current, and wind conditions.

Other Wave Terms

A group of waves approaching the shore is called a *set*. The number of waves within each set can vary, as can the size and shape of each individual wave. A much larger wave in a set is called a *rogue wave*. Rogue waves—caused by an anomaly in energy at the point the swell originated—have been known to be several times larger than any other wave in a swell. Their existence emphasizes the importance for the need to stay alert while surfing, because they can catch a lot of people off guard both in the water and on shore. Luckily for oceanfront residents, the truly massive rogue waves are relatively rare.

Downtime between wave sets is called a *lull*. The length of a lull can vary considerably, depending on the *consistency* of the swell. A very consistent swell may have waves breaking regularly with lulls varying from a few minutes to not at all. When larger waves are breaking regularly with good shape, the surf is said to be *pumping*. On such days, many surfers welcome the occasional lull in order to recover. In most areas, swells commonly contain periodic lulls of up to several minutes.

The place where surfers wait for waves is called the *lineup*, and it's determined by where the peak of the wave has been. It's helpful to use landmarks on shore to give yourself a reference point for where you want to be when you paddle back out to the lineup. If you're too far left or right, you run the risk of not catching the wave at the peak. If you're too far *outside*—too far from shore—it might be too difficult to catch the wave. If you're too far *inside*—too close to shore—the wave might break before you have a chance to catch it.

Another pitfall to being too far inside is that you increase your odds of being caught off guard by a *cleanup set*. Cleanup sets are usually larger outside sets that close out before anyone can get to them. Surfers caught just inside of where the waves break are said to be in the *impact zone*. The impact zone is sometimes a dangerous place to be, especially when the waves are big. Large amounts of whitewater can make it tough to paddle back outside or even hold your position. Some surf spots have shallow, treacherous areas known as *boneyards* that can make the impact zone even more unpleasant!

GEAR

Before we get to the subject of actually riding waves we need to discuss the gear associated with the sport. I highly recommend visiting your local surf shop and talking to someone who's actually used any gear you're interested in getting. They should be able to help you choose the best product for your goals, needs, wants, and abilities. It's important to be aware of what's available because the right equipment can enhance both your performance and your stoke!

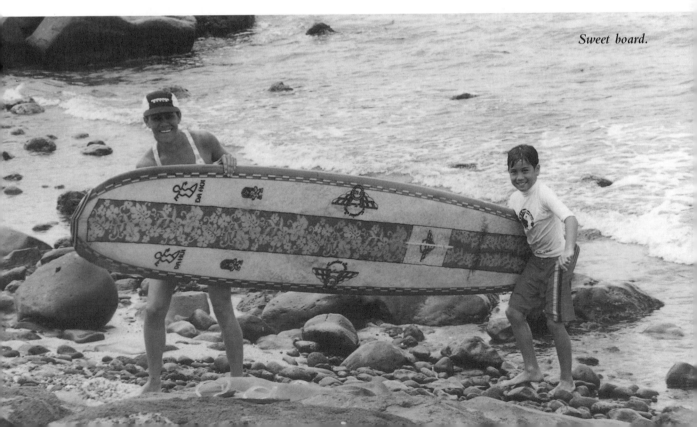

Sweet board.

Boards

Surfboards come in many different designs, with a variety of bottom, width, and rocker combinations. The combination that will be best for you depends on your weight, ability, style, and the types of waves you're riding. Different breaks require different equipment, so many avid surfers have what is known as a *quiver* of *sticks*—a variety of different boards. Surfboard preference is extremely individual. As you progress in the sport, you'll develop a better understanding of equipment and what your specific needs are. An experienced *shaper*, one who shapes boards, can work with you to create a truly *custom* or individualized board. It's best, however, for surfers and shapers to build a stick that's functional rather than conforming to the fads of the industry.

Design

Basic surfboard designs include shortboards, fun-shapes, longboards, big-wave boards and big-wave tow-in boards. Boards within each category share similar dimension and shape characteristics that make them better suited for a particular type of surfing. Keep in mind that what follows are generalizations and that surfboard designs within each grouping can vary significantly. A multitude of factors influence a board's design, such as the intended surfer's weight, ability, style, and the size and shape of the waves ridden.

Dimensions

Surfboards dimensions are usually written on the bottom of the board.

The first number is usually the board's length in feet and inches. The second number is usually the nose width of the board—the width as measured 1 foot from the *nose* or front section of the board. The third number is usually the middle width of the board, while the fourth

Basic Boards

Design	Description	Approximate Length
Shortboard	Short and oblong with a pointed nose	6'–7'
Funshape	Midsized board between a long and short board	7'–9'
Longboard	Long and relatively straight with a round nose	9'-plus
Big-wave board (aka gun or rhino chaser)	Long and skinny at the nose and tail	9'-plus
Big-wave tow-in board	Similar to a shortboard but with foot straps	7'–8'

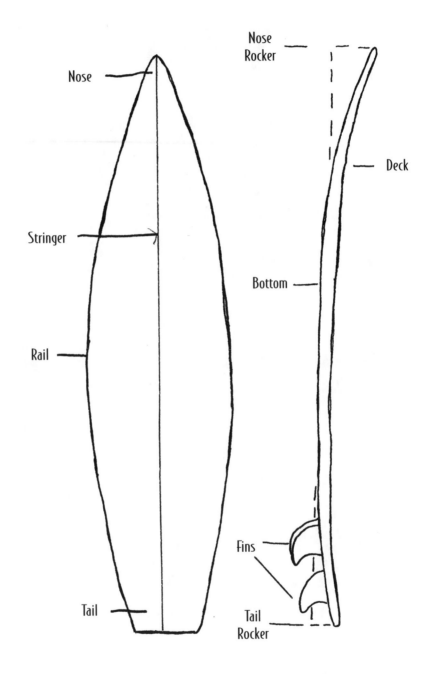

Nose

Nose
Rocker

Deck

Stringer

Bottom

Rail

Fins

Tail

Tail
Rocker

Anatomy of a surf board.

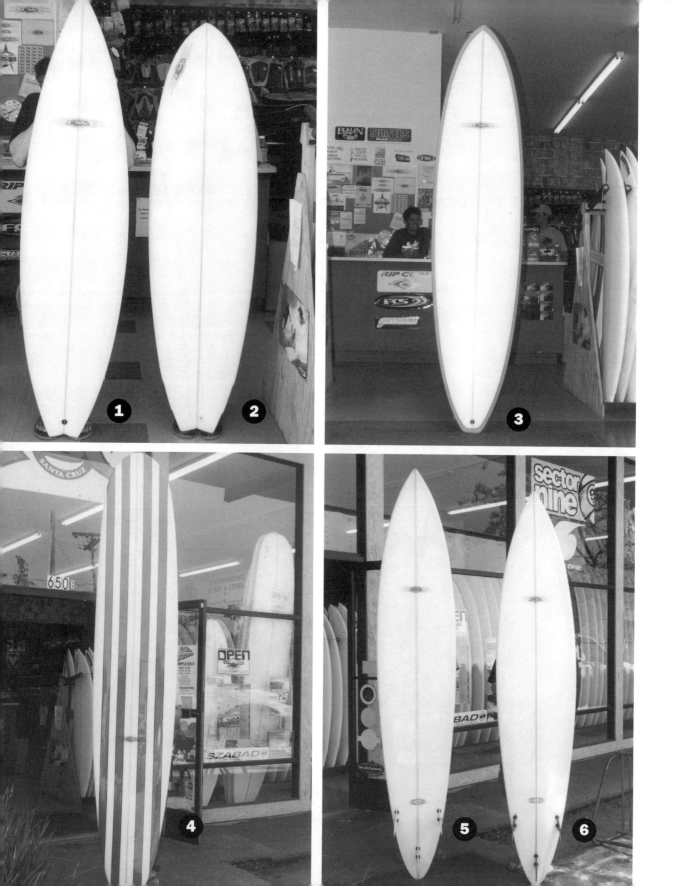

Typical Board Dimensions

Design	Length	Nose	Width	Tail	Thickness
Shortboard	6'6"	11"	19"	12"	2½"
Funshape	7'6"	13"	20"	14"	2¾"
Longboard	9'6"	18"	23"	14"	3"
Big-wave	10'	11"	21"	10"	3"
Tow-in	7'	16"	22"	17"	2"

number is the tail width, as measured 1 foot from the *tail* or rear portion of the board. The fifth number is usually the thickness of the board in the middle. Some shapers write these dimensions in a different order on the board, but you can figure it out pretty easily.

Characteristics

Boards differ in any number of ways. Here are some that you should be familiar with.

- *Materials.* The majority of surfboards are made of fiberglass and foam with a balsa wood stringer. Other common materials include carbon, graphite, Kevlar, and plastic. Beginner's boards are often made with spongy foam on the top and plastic on the bottom. The materials used affect board weight, performance, and durability.
- *Blank.* A blank is the generic piece of foam from which a surfboard is shaped. Blanks are purchased by shapers in a variety of different sizes, depending on what type of board they intend to shape.
- *Outline.* The outline refers to the outer shape or silhouette of a surfboard. It can give you a general idea of how the board will perform in the water.
- *Stringer thickness.* The stringer is the thin strip of wood, usually balsa, in the middle of the board that affects strength and rigidity. Some boards have very thick or multiple stringers.
- *Rocker.* This term refers to how much the board curves at the nose and tail. The amount of rocker in the board can affect its carving or turning performance, because it shortens the board's natural arc. Shorter boards generally have more rocker than longer boards—they're designed for shorter-radius turns. Rocker also affects board speed. A board with more rocker

Opposite page:
1. *6'5" channel-bottom swallow tail.*
2. *6'1" fish double-wing swallow tail.*
3. *7'10" hybrid.*
4. *10' longboard.*
5. *9' gun with ½" stringer.*
6. *8'6" gun.*

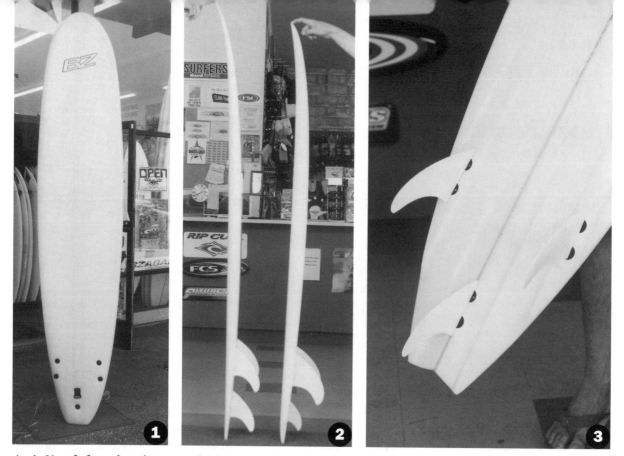

1. *A 9' soft foam board is great for learning.* 2. *Profile of two shortboards: Notice the rocker.*
3. *A channel-bottom swallow tail thruster.*

will have less of its bottom touching the water at any given time. This decrease in surface area equates to less speed.

- *Rail shape.* The sides or turning edges of the surfboard are known as *rails*. They can vary from thick and round to thin and tapered. Rail shape can affect buoyancy and consequently the ability to catch waves. The shape of the rails also influences carving performance, because it helps determine how the board responds when it is put on edge.

- *Deck.* The deck is the top of the board, where a surfer stands. On fiberglass boards, this is where wax is rubbed on or traction pads are applied to prevent slipping.

- *Bottom.* The shape of a board's bottom or underside can affect performance. Bottom

shape can vary from relatively flat, like that of a traditional longboard, to concave, like that of a V-bottom-shaped shortboard. Some boards have grooves in the bottom called channels. The angles at which the channels are shaped affect the way water flows under the board, which in turn will alter the board's performance.

- *Concave.* How concave the bottom of a board is can affect responsiveness and speed. Boards vary from slightly to deeply concave, and from single to triple concave.

- *Tail shape.* The shape of the board's tail can vary considerably, ranging from straight to squash, split, swallow, or fish tail. This shape affects how the board will finish a turn.

- *Flex.* Incorporating flex into surfboards is the future of design. Traditionally, boards have been rigid and require the surfer to make adjustments to the constantly changing terrain of a wave. These days, however, some boards are being made to flex much the same way a snowboard does. Such boards have an inner core that consists of carbon graphite and woven glass fiber that are melded together. Surrounding the core is shapable foam, which is then covered with urethane.

• *Graphics.* Anything goes. Graphics should not affect board performance.

Fins

Fins are placed near the tail of the board to provide stability and control, as well as assisting in turning. Some surfboards have fins permanently adhered to them, while others allow for fins to be removed. The removable system gives you a chance to experiment with different types of fins, depending on your preference, style, ability, and conditions.

Types of Fins

Numerous designs, shapes, sizes, and materials are used for fins. The shape and size of the fins will affect how a surfboard performs. Placement is important, too: Fins that are placed farther forward loosen up a board and shorten its turning arc. Also note that the angle at which fins are placed on the board will affect its responsiveness and speed.

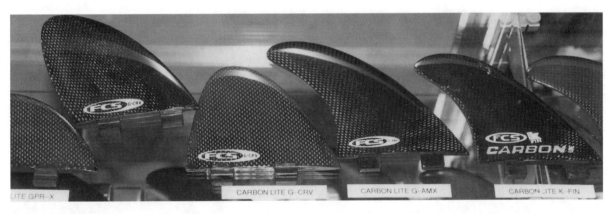

Various fin designs.

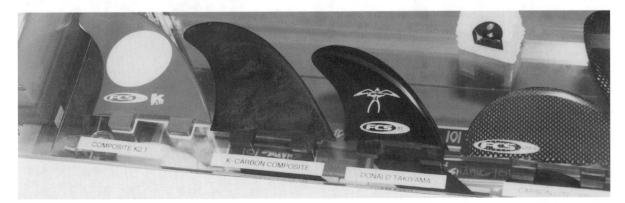

Number of Fins

- *Single fin.* A single fin is one, usually large, middle fin; it's generally seen only on longboards. Some longboarders now use a large single fin that has a hollow tube running through it, which helps lengthen the duration of their noserides.
- *Double fin or twin.* This configuration uses two medium-sized fins and is found on all types of boards.
- *Tri-fin or thruster.* In this very popular fin configuration, one small to medium-sized fin is placed in the middle and two fins of the same size or smaller are placed on either side of it. The thruster-fin configuration can be found on all types of boards.

- *Quad fin or twinzer.* The twinzer consists of a set of two relatively small fins on each side. This can be used on all types of boards.
- *Five fin.* The five-fin configuration is a twinzer with a small to medium-sized middle fin. It's usually found only on shortboards.

Wet Suits

A wet suit is a snug-fitting, neoprene suit most commonly worn by surfers at cold-water breaks. Wet suits allow you to stay warmer longer by trapping water in the suit, which is then warmed by your body. They're made in a variety of styles, sizes, thicknesses, and materials. A full wet suit covers the torso, arms, and legs, with the neoprene usually thicker in the torso and thinner at

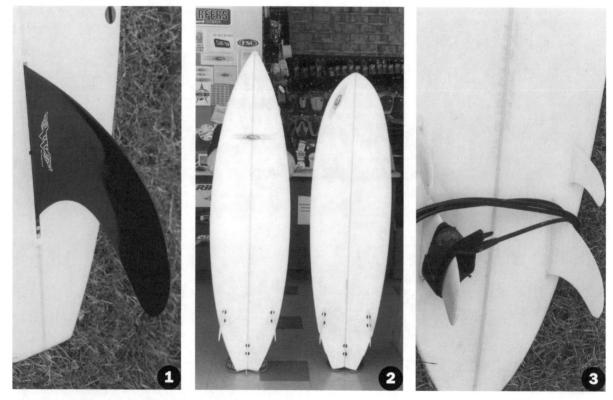

1. Longboard single fin. 2. Shortboard thrusters. 3. Twinzer.

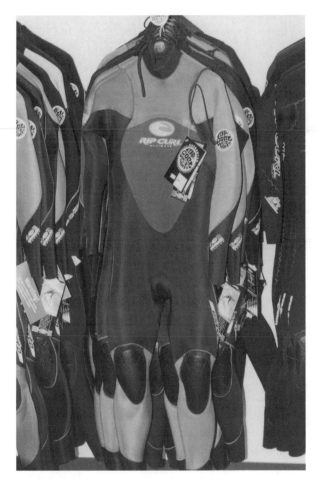

Wet suits.

the extremities. The thicker the wet suit, the warmer it is. Like most apparel, wet suits are made in different sizes to accommodate surfers' various heights and shapes. A suit should be snug but still allow you to move freely.

The most common wet-suit thickness what's known as a 3/2 (3 millimeters thick in the torso, 2 millimeters in the arms and legs). In the winter, many surfers at cold-water breaks use a 4/3 (4 millimeters in the torso, 3 in the extremities). A spring suit has short sleeves and legs and is most commonly a 2/1 (2 millimeters in the

torso and 1 millimeter in the limbs). There are various other style and thickness combinations, as well as top- or bottom-only suits.

Wet suits also differ in terms of the materials used. Some suits are made with materials that allow for greater freedom of movement. Others are reinforced at the seams to provide extra warmth and durability.

A dry suit is completely waterproof and is generally only worn when surfing extremely cold-water breaks. The suit forms a tight seal at the openings and has a waterproof zipper.

Leashes

The leash is what connects you to your board. A securing string is attached to a plug found on the board's deck, near the tail. This string is looped so that Velcro can fasten a piece of webbing called a rail saver to it. The rail saver is then attached to a urethane cord that has swivels at either end to prevent the cord from getting twisted. The opposite end of the cord is attached to an ankle strap that is fastened with Velcro around your back foot.

Leashes are made in different lengths depending on the size of the board, the size of the waves, and the preference of the surfer. You may choose to put an 8-foot leash on your shortboard and a 12-foot leash on a big-wave board. In areas that have a lot of kelp, it's important to check your leash regularly while surfing to make sure it's free of debris. A leash is a must for beginning surfers and surfing in big waves. It should not, however, be taken for granted: it's still imperative that you attempt to hang on to your board at all times. A speeding board can easily become a projectile, even on a leash. Many advanced long-boarders will surf without a leash when the waves are relatively small, allowing more freedom in walking around the board.

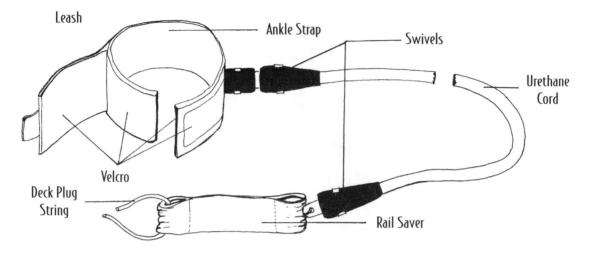

Surfboard leash.

Out of the water, it's best to wrap the leash around the tail of the board and secure it to a fin. This will help keep the Velcro from collecting sand as well as preventing incidental tripping or snagging.

Wax and Traction Pads

Wax is rubbed onto the deck of traditional fiberglass boards to provide traction. Unlike other dynamic balance sports such as skiing, snowboarding, and wakeboarding, the only boards to which you strap your feet are big-wave tow-in boards. As a result, it's imperative that your feet be able to grip the surface of the board. First, you apply a base coat of wax, over which you rub either a warm- or cold-water wax of your preference. The goal is to create small humps of wax on the board that will provide a nonslip surface. Before every surf session a thin layer of wax can be applied to the existing layer to keep the deck tacky. After a few sessions, the wax may start to get dirty and lose its ability to adhere to the board. Thus, it's important to periodically scrape your board and apply a fresh coat of wax. Leaving the board deck-side up in the sun for a few minutes will make it easier to use a plastic ice scraper or something similar to clear the old wax. The foam-top boards that are made for beginners don't require wax.

On fiberglass boards, traction pads can be used in place of wax. These pads adhere to the deck of the board and are made of durable rubber. Numerous types are made for all kinds of boards. The most common traction pad, more often seen on shortboards, is applied to the rear of the board to provide traction for your rear foot. You can also find very thin traction pads that have graphics on them. These are commonly applied only to the nose of longboards.

Other Equipment

- *Nose guards.* Nose guards are rubber strips used to cover the tips of surfboards. They have

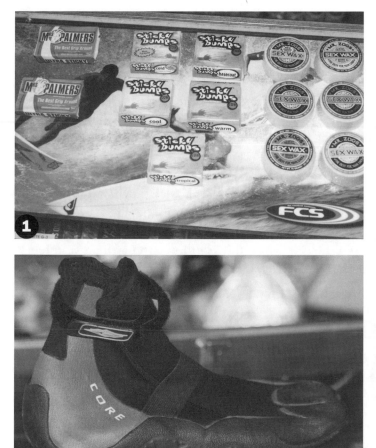

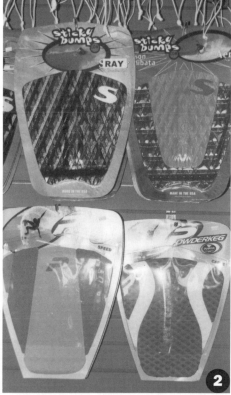

1. Surfboard wax.
2. Traction pads.
3. Surf bootie.

a very strong adhesive backing and are easy to apply. Nose guards are advisable, especially for pointed shortboards. All too many surfers have been injured as a result of getting speared by their board, or someone else's! Similar guards can also be applied to the fin(s) of the board for added safety and have little or no effect on the board's performance characteristics.

- *Booties.* Booties are rubber-soled neoprene shoes worn by many surfers at cold-water surf spots. In areas where sharp coral, rocks, or sea urchins are found, some surfers will also wear booties to prevent cuts and abrasions. A majority of the booties on the market today have tacky soles with grooves in them that help deliver pretty good traction. Still, you'll find that many surfers prefer the feel they get for the board with bare feet regardless of the air or water temperature.

- *Gloves.* Some surfers wear neoprene gloves at cold-water breaks for winter warmth. Occasionally, you'll see a surfer wearing webbed gloves to aid in paddling.

- *Hoods.* Another item used for warmth during

the winter months at cold-water surf spots is the neoprene hood. Hoods can be especially helpful in minimizing heat loss, since most body heat is lost through our heads.

- *Helmets.* Some surfers wear helmets for protection at shallow or otherwise dangerous breaks. Like hoods, helmets can also aid in maintaining warmth.
- *Rash guards.* Rash guards are short- or long-sleeved tops worn by some surfers and are usually made of Lycra or very thin neoprene. They are most commonly used at warm-water surf spots to minimize chafing from the board while paddling and as protection from the sun. Some surfers also wear a rash guard under their wet suit at cold-water surf spots to serve as an additional layer of warmth.
- *Board shorts.* Board shorts are durable shorts worn while surfing in warm water. Usually longer than traditional shorts, they dry very quickly. Board shorts are made without open pockets in order to prevent water from flowing inside while you paddle.
- *Sunscreen.* We all know how important it is to protect our skin from the sun's damaging rays. While surfing, it's advisable to choose a sunscreen that's both waterproof and sweatproof.
- *Hats.* Some surfers wear a hat or visor while

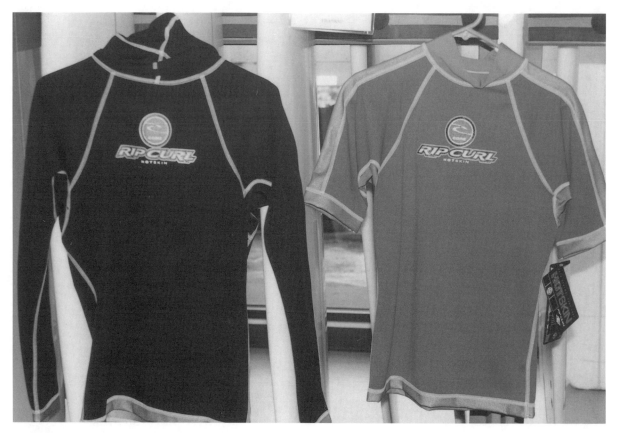

Rash guards.

surfing relatively small waves. Hats can help keep the sun off your face and protect your eyes but are not advised for novice surfers, who will probably find their heads under water periodically.

- *Board bags.* Board bags are used to protect surfboards while traveling. They come in numerous sizes to accommodate different lengths and numbers of boards. Some bags are made of reflective material that will help keep the board cool while it sits in the sun. Other bags are heavily padded to protect the board from airport baggage handlers. No matter how well-padded a board bag is, however, it's advisable to encase your board in bubble wrap before you fly.

- *Board cases.* These cases are made of durable, lightweight plastic to provide additional travel protection.

- *Board socks.* Board socks are cotton or terry-cloth covers used to protect boards in daily use, helping to keep them clean and cool. They also serve as protection when boards are stacked on a roof rack or in storage.

- *Roof racks.* These racks are used to fasten surf-boards to the tops of vehicles. The two main types are hard and soft. Hard racks are usually made of metal and are designed to stay on the vehicle more or less permanently. They consist of four posts or towers that attach to the roof, plus two bars that run the width of the vehicle. Foam pads are then placed on the bars, and straps are used to tie the boards down. Avid surfers who transport their boards frequently prefer hard racks. Soft racks are simply foam pads with webbing running through them. The webbing is long enough to run through the inside of the vehicle, and other straps are used to hold the board down. Soft

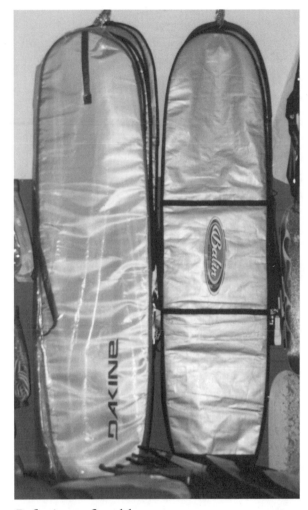

Reflective surfboard bags.

racks are less expensive and more portable, making them ideal for traveling.

- *Ding repair kits.* At some point in almost every board's lifetime, it incurs a *ding*—a puncture or dent. In the case of fiberglass-and-foam boards, dings through the fiberglass need to be repaired to prevent the inner foam from becoming waterlogged. Minor dings can be taken care of by buying a (relatively inexpensive) ding repair kit, which generally consists of resin, hardener, fiberglass cloth, filler, sandpaper, mixing sticks, a sanding block, and instructions. In the case of major damage, such as *delaminating* (when the fiberglass separates from the foam core), it's best to leave the work to an experienced board repair specialist. This will cost more but also increase your chances for a successful repair.

Equipment Care

Taking care of your equipment is relatively easy and can definitely prolong its useful life. There are three major rules of surf equipment care:

- *Rule 1: Rinse off everything that's been in salt water with fresh water.* This should be done as soon as possible after surfing. Over time, salt water will damage just about any material you can think of.
- *Rule 2: Avoid leaving things in the sun.* The sun will also damage just about any material you can think of. It's best to dry wet suits and other apparel by hanging them in a shady place.
- *Rule 3: Repair board dings immediately.* Every time you surf a board that's dinged, you increase the probability that the damage will require a major repair.

It's Up to You

Equipment innovations have done a great deal for the sport of surfing over the years. And it's easy to get caught up in the quest for the newest and most unusual gear. As you progress in the sport, you'll be able to better appreciate subtle differences in equipment. Advanced surfers develop gear preferences based on feel and performance needs. It's difficult to make generalizations about what board or fin designs will work best for a particular break, because so many individual factors affect performance. For example,

your weight, strength, power, style, and technique can all affect your preferred gear for a certain shape, size, and speed of wave. As a result, most avid surfers collect a virtual arsenal of surfboards and accessories. As with most sports, however, superior equipment can do only so much for your performance. Often the intermediate surfer will look for answers to technique shortcomings by making equipment changes. Keep in mind that athletes like Kelly Slater can surf circles around almost everyone at your home break with a board abandoned in a Dumpster. In other words, there's no substitute for skill, fitness, and overall athleticism.

RESPECT

The golden rule in surf etiquette is to show respect. That means respect for your fellow surfers as well as for the environment. As our planet and surf spots become more crowded, it becomes increasingly important that we surfers not act as if we're the only one in the water.

Every surf spot has its *locals*—surfers who live near and surf a break on a regular basis. Locals in certain areas are very protective of what they consider to be "their" break. For example, a multitude of great surfers reside on and visit the Hawaiian island of Oahu. The locals use the Hawaiian word *haole*, meaning "nonlocals" to refer to people they don't recognize. The North Shore of Oahu has become especially popular, and it's rare that a respectful visiting surfer will be hassled by a local. The local surfers on the West Shore of the island, on the other hand, will make their presence known to haoles. Luckily, aggression or violence is usually only provoked at such spots if visitors show disrespect.

The weekend.

Bottom line: It's wise to be overly respectful when visiting someone else's home break!

Out of the water, it's a good idea to be friendly toward your fellow surfers. Be courteous, lend people wax, and never litter. Most surfers are pretty easygoing, but don't expect to be cut any slack if you act like a jerk.

In the water, there are three rules to live by:

- *Rule 1:* Don't be a wave hog.
- *Rule 2:* Don't drop in on others.
- *Rule 3:* Don't endanger others.

Everything that follows falls under one of the three main rules of etiquette.

Lineups

The *lineup*, or the area where surfers wait for waves, is subject to rule 1. When the waves are consistent and there aren't too many surfers, there usually isn't a problem with the lineup.

We're Not the Only Ones Having Fun Out There!

Sea otters can be routinely seen bobbing over incoming swell while they bask in the sun and play in the waves.

Seals seem to enjoy swimming under speeding surfboards, bumping dangling feet, and playfully tugging on surfers' leashes.

Pelicans are known to fly single file just inches above the water and close enough to the surf to feel the spray from breaking waves.

Dolphins have long been known as one of the most intelligent creatures in the sea. There have been numerous sightings of them bodysurfing, both alone and in groups.

After you've caught a wave, you paddle back to the lineup and wait your turn for another wave. When it's crowded and waves are few and far between, however, surfers tend to be a little more aggressive. A large group of surfers in the lineup is referred to as a *pack*, and it can be a dangerous place for a novice surfer on a crowded day. When good waves are rare, it's common to see many surfers paddling for a wave. This free-for-all approach can lead to surfers colliding and tempers flaring. On some such weekend days, the takeoff area for a wave can resemble the mass start of a triathlon—except a wall of water is pushing these individuals, and each possesses a potential projectile weapon!

Lining up or sitting in a bad spot is also a no-no. If you're waiting for waves too far left or right of the peak, you stand a good chance of not being able to catch a wave. No one will hassle you for doing that. On the other hand, if you're waiting for waves too far inside or too close to the beach, you might end up being in an approaching surfer's way. This is known as being in a bad spot. Sometimes beginners will rest inside on their way back out to the lineup, unaware that they could be putting themselves in a dangerous situation. Or they might line up inside their fellow surfers, hoping to catch smaller waves that break closer to shore. Surfers who choose such a position do so at their own risk and need to be very alert and prepared to paddle extremely hard to get out of the way. If you're tired, the best place to rest is on the beach. The second best place to rest or sit, so that you won't be in anyone's way, is far left or right of the lineup.

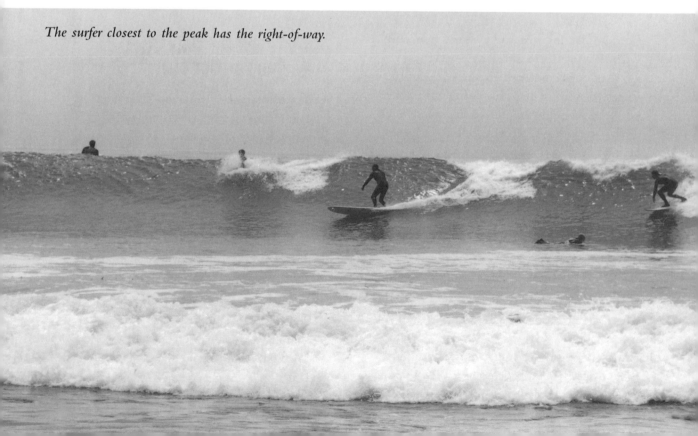

The surfer closest to the peak has the right-of-way.

Right-of-Way

Determining right-of-way on a wave is very simple: The surfer closest to the peak of the wave has the right-of-way. This means that if you're on a wave breaking from left to right, and you're turning right, you need to allow a surfer who is overtaking you to have the wave. Sometimes surfers will agree to share waves when it's crowded—but never assume this to be the case.

When two surfers take off at the peak of a wave that can be surfed either left or right, the easiest thing for them to do is turn away from one another once they're standing. It's customary in such situations to ask which way the other surfer intends to go before you paddle for the wave.

Dropping In

The most important thing to know in terms of etiquette is that you don't *drop in* on or *cut off* other surfers. These terms both refer to catching a wave in front of surfers who are closer to the breaking part of the wave. Because they are closer to the peak, they have the right-of-way and are more than likely going to overtake you. Dropping in on them may result in you interfering with their ride or causing a collision. As I mentioned, surfers at some spots don't mind sharing waves on a crowded day. In many cases, however, dropping in is a good way to make enemies and start fights. Always look toward the peak of the wave to make sure no one else has already taken off. If you accidentally drop in on folks, turn out of the wave immediately. Apologize as they go by; when you see them again in the lineup, you might want to apologize again in case they didn't hear you the first time.

Paddling Out

When you're paddling out to the lineup, try to

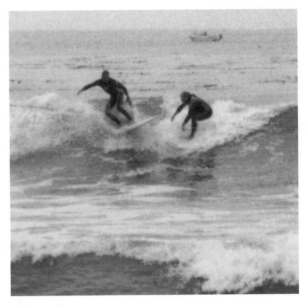

Near collision.

stay clear of other surfers. If possible, paddle around the breaking waves so that you can avoid interfering with another surfer's ride. Paddling around the break is especially important when it's crowded or the waves are very consistent. If you've ever been skiing or snowboarding on a crowded day at a resort, you've probably witnessed collisions between riders. Differences in speed, abilities, and people stopping below knolls where they can't be seen by overtaking riders are common causes of such mishaps. Similarly, avoid paddling directly into a rider's path or waiting for waves just inside of other surfers where they'll have to turn to avoid hitting you. Ideally, the area where surfers are riding waves should remain clear. Surfers who have just finished a ride and surfers who have unsuccessfully paddled for a wave should paddle back to the line-up around the breaking waves. If everyone followed this practice, "traffic" would flow in a circular pattern; paddling surfers and riding surfers would never meet in a head-on collision. In the event that you find yourself in a surfer's path, paddle toward the whitewater. This will give the approaching surfer a clear path to the unbroken part of the wave. If there are multiple surfers approaching you on the same wave, your only option may be to "thread the needle," or paddle between two of them. In this case, paddle as fast as you can in the hope that you can get by without disrupting someone's ride. Still, if you're aware of your surroundings, you don't sit in obviously bad spots, and you hustle, paddling out should be a piece of cake!

Falling

When you're falling, make every possible attempt to grab the rails or any other part of the board to prevent it from hitting someone else. The term *grabbing rail* refers to holding on to the sides

of the board. This is especially important for beginners who are trying to paddle out or who tend to fall off the board often. A surfboard can quickly turn into a projectile if it's allowed to speed through the whitewater. At the very least, grab the leash immediately and yank the board toward you. Even if you don't see anyone in the surfboard's path, it's wise to always stay in control of your board. And when it's crowded, it's imperative that you try to foresee and avoid situations that might result in you falling and losing your board. For example, if a wave is closing out, try to turn out of it, or simply drop down on the board and drag both legs in the water until the board stops.

Bailing is the act of diving off a surfboard, usually in order to avoid being punished by a wave. When it's not crowded and a wave has closed out, many surfers will bail or jump off the

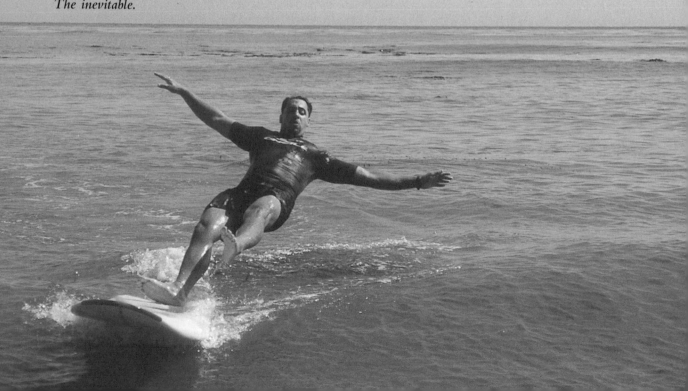

The inevitable.

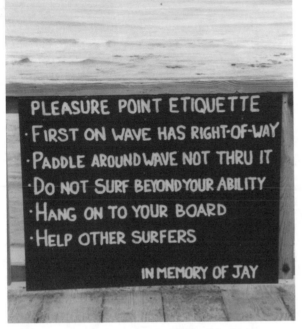

Surfing etiquette in memory of Jay Moriarty, a Santa Cruz surfer, who died young.

board and over the whitewater to end a ride. This is fine—*if* you have a strong leash and are certain no one is in the board's path. It's a bad habit for beginners to adopt, though: On a crowded or big day, jumping off your board can result in serious injury. Learn how to control your board at all times.

What We Do in Life . . .

Overall, use common sense when you're in the water. The last thing you want to do is sour a sweet session by hurting someone or making folks angry. The more people there are in the water and the bigger the waves, the more important it is that you remain alert and watch out for others.

When you think of surfing etiquette, think of the following quote from the film *The Gladiator*: "What we do in life echoes in eternity."

Pay It Forward

Remember that movie *Pay It Forward*, where the kid wants to change the world by doing something nice for three strangers? The idea was that if the three strangers in turn did something nice for three more strangers, and so on, eventually the world would be a better place. Well, the world of surfing needs that kind of mentality. There are no referees or other figures of authority out in the waves in which we play. We are responsible for regulating ourselves. If you let someone closer to the peak have the "wave of the session" or you take the whitewater when you're paddling out, that surfer is more likely to return the favor to someone else and, most importantly, to you!

SURFING 101

The ancient Hawaiians believed that people could achieve greatness only after establishing a balance among themselves, their fellow humans, and nature. In much the same way, I offer that you cannot become a truly great surfer until you have struck a balance among you, your fellow surfers, and the ocean. In other words, surfing is more than just jumping on a board. For some, it can be a metaphor for life. To truly experience all that surfing has to offer, be prepared to show a little humility as well as strive to continuously learn and grow as both a surfer and an individual. As Kahlil Gibran once wrote, "Drink the water as if it were drinking you."

The best conditions for inexperienced surfers to refine their skills are days when the waves are well shaped, hip high, and just crumble over. Small, mushy waves work fine for beginners. All you really need in order to learn how to surf on a longboard is a wave just strong enough to propel you. Also, a place with a sandy bottom

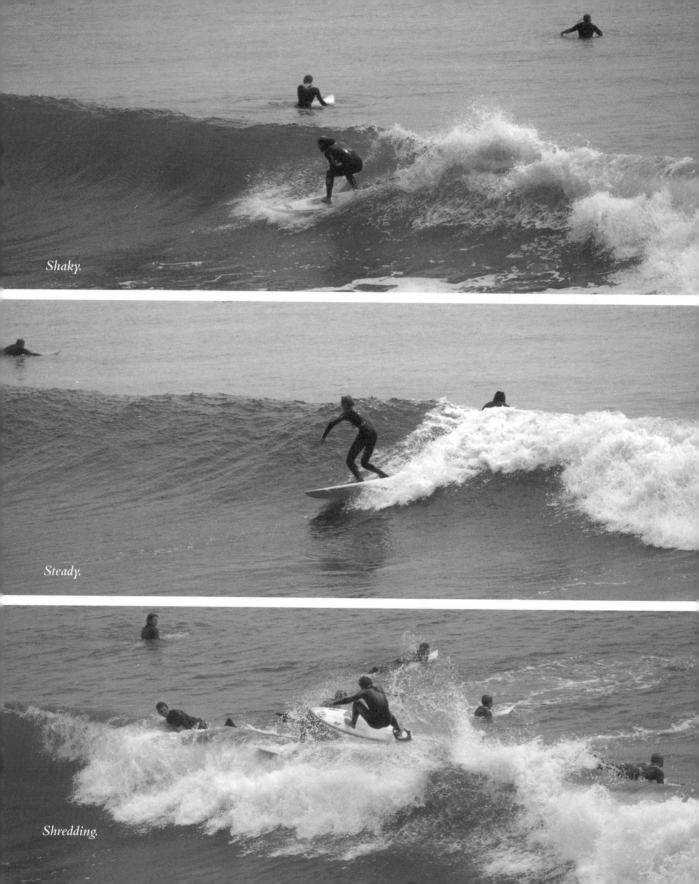

Shaky.

Steady.

Shredding.

is a great place to start out. You don't want to be around rocks, cliffs, or too many people as a novice, because you can expect to part ways with your board often!

Learning how to surf can be a frustrating endeavor. It can be painful for the deconditioned and humiliating for the disrespectful. Novice surfers are referred to as *kooks* for their inexperience in the water. It's a rite of passage of sorts, and most advanced surfers will usually give a beginner the benefit of the doubt. Still, most experienced surfers also expect you to learn quickly and not make the same mistake twice. Above all, keep in mind that knowledge and experience are power. Try to become a student of the sport just as you are (hopefully) a student of life.

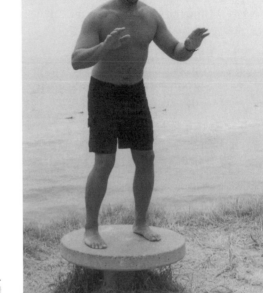

Ready position, front view.

Basic Body Position

The basic body position on a surfboard is what I refer to as the "ready" position. It's a stance that allows you to react in every direction or plane of movement and can be seen in a variety of sports—skiing, snowboarding, tennis, football, and basketball, to name just a few. The ready position involves standing with your knees somewhat bent, each one aligned with the middle of the foot. Your feet are shoulder width apart; distribute your weight a little more on the balls of your feet than on your heels. Your hips should be slightly lowered, your spine in a neutral position and angled slightly forward. Head and chest are up; shoulders and hips level; hands in front of the body. This stance helps keep your center of gravity low and makes it easier to quickly recenter and balance dynamically.

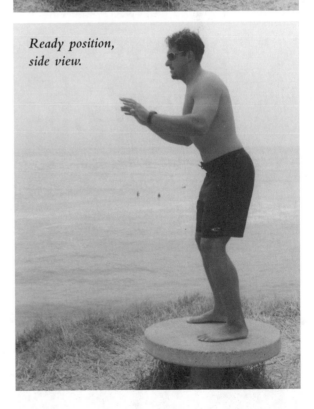

Ready position, side view.

Biomechanics

Biomechanics refers to the joint positions and muscles used for any movement. The ideal biomechanics for any movement puts you in the strongest, safest, and most powerful position. Learning the correct biomechanics for any sport is the key to optimal performance. You *can* perform a variety of movements in sport and life with poor mechanics—but your efficiency, strength, power, balance, stability, and ability to prevent injury are all compromised. For example, throwing a ball, swinging a racquet, or throwing a punch can all be done by using mostly your arms. If you instead "lead with your hips" or initiate torso rotation with the lower body, however, you can get your weight into it and throw the ball farther, generate more racquet speed, and punch harder. As a result, you've not only enhanced your performance but also decreased the forces incurred by your shoulder joint.

The same holds true for surfing. You *can* stand on the board with your legs locked, your spine bent over at the waist, and your hands behind you. If you do so, however, your center of gravity will be high and forward. Thus, your control of the board and ability to react to changes in speed or direction will be greatly reduced, and your chance of injury amplified.

Weight Transfer

Like any sport that requires you to remain balanced in a dynamic environment, surfing demands the ability to transfer your weight constantly. At slower speeds these weight transfers tend to be subtle. At higher speeds they can be powerful and aggressive movements. In surfing you transfer weight from heel to toe, side to side, and rotationally in order to remain balanced and to perform various maneuvers. The ready position helps you make all these weight transfers quickly and easily.

Paddling

Paddling a surfboard requires strength, stability,

Paddling Tips

1. Get centered on the board.
2. Keep your head and chest up.
3. Keep your legs together.
4. Cup your hands.
5. Relax your shoulders.

and practice. For the avid surfer, paddling becomes a relatively effortless skill. For the novice, paddling can be frustrating and painful. It helps if you're relatively fit and accustomed to strenuous exercise. It can definitely be a workout until you become more efficient.

1. *Get centered on the board.* Paddling a surfboard is a lot easier if the board can glide through the water. In order to decrease resistance while you paddle, it's important to center your weight both side to side and front to back. If your weight is too far off to one side, the rail of the board will be under water, slowing you down. If your weight is too far back, the nose of the board will be up in the air and the board will *stall*—that is, it'll lose speed as a result of pushing a lot of water. From the side a stalling surfboard looks like it's "popping a wheelie." If your weight is too far forward, the board will *pearl*. Pearling refers to the nose of a moving surfboard submerging. Both stalling and pearling affect your board's *trim*. A board that is in trim is level and can carry more speed.

2. *Keep your head and chest up.* Most novice surfers have a great deal of difficulty keeping their chests up while lying facedown on a surfboard. It requires a great deal of back extensor strength and endurance. It is, however, the key to powerful paddling. When your chest is up, you're able to pull water more easily because your shoulders are in a stronger position. In other words, you have a greater biomechanical advantage when paddling with your chest off the board. Keeping your head up will help you keep your shoulders relaxed and your stroke fluid, while also keeping you alert and safer.

3. *Keep your legs together.* Efficient paddling requires that the board remain as stable as possible to maximize glide through the water. If

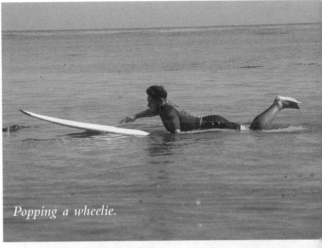

Popping a wheelie.

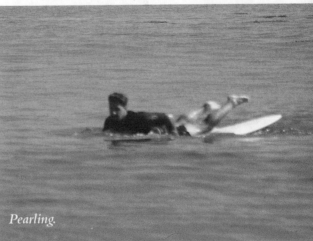

Pearling.

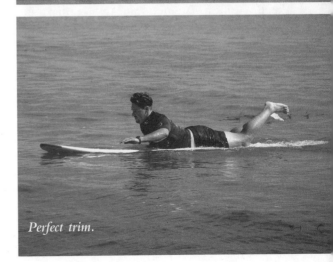

Perfect trim.

your legs are moving around, it takes more energy to keep the board level. And if your feet are dangling in the water, you're creating more drag and ultimately more work for yourself.

4. *Cup your hands.* Cupping your hands the way swimmers do will allow you to capture more water and paddle faster. You can also employ some swimming arm strokes, such as the S stroke. This involves drawing an S through the water during your paddle stroke. When done correctly, this technique can increase your board speed significantly.

5. *Relax your shoulders.* When you pull your arm through the water, you should focus on using the muscles best designed for the job. In paddling, this happens to be the latissimus dorsi (lats). The lats attach at the back of the upper arm and fan down the back. As a result, they are great for any movement that involves pulling. When you relax your shoulders, or more specifically your trapezius muscles, you make it easier for the shoulder to retract, allowing the lat to do more work. Besides making your paddle stroke more fluid and efficient, relaxing your shoulders can help keep you from fatiguing quickly and make it easier to keep your head and chest up.

Paddling Out

Paddling out to where the waves break can be challenging and sometimes dangerous. You should never paddle out when the waves are too big for your ability or conditioning. During a storm swell, waves can be large and very frequent, leaving little downtime or rest for the inexperienced or out-of-shape surfer. Watch how other surfers are getting out to the lineup. You want to pick the easiest and safest way out past

the whitewater. As a novice, you'll want to go out on days that are small and not intimidating. Small days will also give you the least resistance for paddling out and will probably be less crowded. If you're having a very difficult time paddling out, you're probably in over your head. It would be wise to take the whitewater in and try again another day.

The following skills will get you through waves that are breaking or have already broken as you paddle out.

- *Use a rip current.* Often the easiest way to get out is to use a rip current, or a low spot in the shore where water is flowing back out to the ocean. A very strong rip can be difficult to exit, however, and inexperienced surfers should stay well clear. When in doubt, stay out! If you do find yourself caught in a rip current, you can paddle parallel to the shore to break free of its force.

- *Pushing up.* If you're paddling out through small, crumbling waves, you can just push your body up off the board and let the wave pass underneath you. This is simply called pushing up. It's important to keep your board pointed straight into the wave when you do this so you don't flip over.

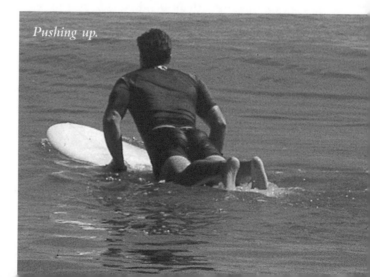
Pushing up.

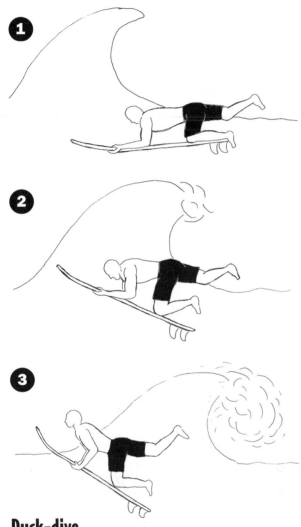

Duck-dive

1. Push the nose of the board under water.
2. Throw your body weight onto the board.
3. Pop up through the back side of the wave.

- *Duck-diving.* Duck-diving is the act of submerging your board to get under a breaking or broken wave. It involves pushing the nose of the board under water and using your body weight to pop it through the other side of the wave. Shortboards are great for this because they're not as buoyant and can easily be pushed under water. Longboards, the type of board you'll be learning on, are much more difficult to manage when paddling out.

- *Slice and duck.* The slice and duck is a technique used to submerge longboards under an oncoming wave. It involves putting the board on edge and then pushing it under water. Once the board is submerged, it's much easier to get it to pop through the back of the wave.

- *Turtle roll.* Another longboard technique used to deal with an oncoming wave or whitewater is the turtle roll. There are different versions of this, but the most common is to grab the board by the rails and wrap your feet around the bottom. You can then flip the board over and let the wave pass by. You shouldn't lose too much ground with this technique as long as you keep the nose of the board down.

Waiting for Waves

Now that you're in the lineup, it's time to get comfortable. As a beginner, you're not going to want to rush into anything. Your first task is to learn how to go from a paddling position to a sitting position on the board. This is fairly easy and will become more natural with practice. You'll notice that it will be easiest to sit comfortably if your legs are dangling directly below you and your weight is centered on the board. Most longboards are very buoyant and will keep you above the water. Just remember to keep the nose of the board pointed toward the oncoming waves. This will allow you to see what's coming and prevent you from getting dumped!

Once you've mastered that, practice turning the board around from your new sitting position. The easiest technique is to "eggbeater" or kick your legs in a circular fashion, like you would if you were treading water. To turn more quickly, keep one hand on the board's rail and push or pull water with the other hand while you egg-beater. Turning around can be made easier if you scoot back on the board. This allows the board's nose to come out of the water and will decrease the amount of resistance you'll have to over-come. At first, this technique might seem awk-ward, but after a while turning the board around should be quick and effortless.

Finally, you'll want to watch other surfers. You'll quickly determine who the more experi-enced surfers out there are. Take notice of how they sit on their boards, paddle, move around in the lineup, turn their boards around, and so on. Try to pay close attention to which waves they pass up and which ones they take. For instance, most experienced surfers can tell whether a wave will close out, or fail to break, as it approaches the lineup. They can also anticipate how a wave will form and break across its length, as well as when and where to move around in the lineup to be at just the right location as the best sets roll through. These senses are acquired through countless surf sessions, and having them can save you a great deal of time and energy. Learn from and emulate the more seasoned surfers—while being careful to not get in their way!

Catching Waves

Catching a wave, also referred to as the *takeoff*, can be more difficult than it might appear. It requires that you be in the right place at the right time, and paddle effectively. Many novice surfers spend several sessions struggling with the takeoff.

1. *Get centered on the board.* Being centered on the board becomes even more important when you're attempting to paddle into a

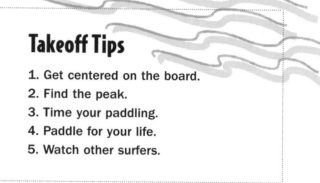

Takeoff Tips

1. **Get centered on the board.**
2. **Find the peak.**
3. **Time your paddling.**
4. **Paddle for your life.**
5. **Watch other surfers.**

wave. If your weight is too far back, the board will stall and you won't generate enough speed to catch the wave. If your weight is too far forward, the nose of the board will become submerged and the board will pearl. Pearling on takeoff usually results in you slid-ing forward and off the board. If you're rock-ing the board from side to side when you're trying to take off, the board will turn and slow—and the wave will pass you over. When you're first starting out, it's best to think about keeping the board as stable as possible and paddling straight into shore.

2. *Find the peak.* Ideally, you want to catch a wave at the *peak*. As I noted earlier, the peak is the breaking part of the wave where it has the most power. Still, when you're first learning, just catching a wave anywhere will suffice. The first couple of times, it's best to simply ride the whitewater in on your stomach and get accustomed to the feeling of being pushed by the wave. Once you're comfortable with this, you can look for an area away from other surfers where the waves are small and practice how to line up. (The lineup, you'll remember, is the area beyond the breaking waves where surfers wait to catch a wave.) Once you've found the peak, you can line it up with a point on the shore so that during a *lull*, or

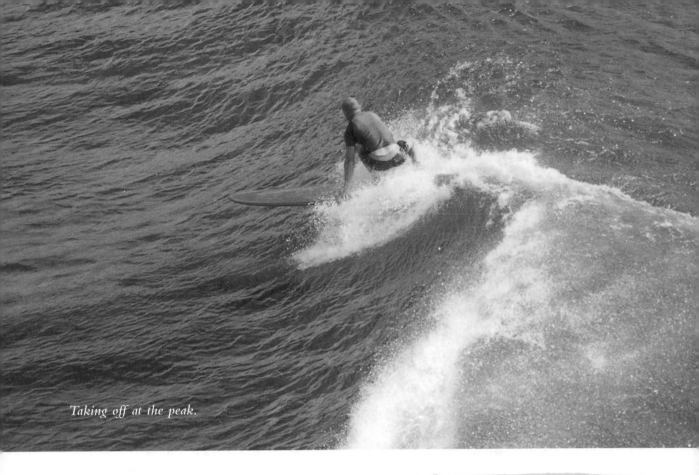

Taking off at the peak.

break between sets of waves, you'll know if you're still in the right place.

But being in the right place in relation to the shore is only half the picture. It's also important to not be too far in or out. If you're too far out or *outside,* the wave won't have enough power to push you. If you're too far in or *inside,* you run the risk of being caught in an area where the waves have already broken. To complicate things further, peaks can shift depending on the swell direction, tide, and current. A break can look very different from day to day or even set to set. This means that you need to be able to identify and anticipate changes in the swell in order to remain in the lineup. For example, if you surf a spot often, you might observe that when you see kelp moving on the horizon you need to move outside. You might also

learn that when the tide is dropping, the peak tends to shift to the right. As a result, the surfers who catch the most waves are usually the most experienced locals.

3. *Time your paddling.* Pearling is most common among novice longboarders who attempt to take off late or when the wave face is steep. A *late takeoff* refers to trying to take off right before the wave breaks. This is usually when the wave face is steepest, and the back of the board gets picked up the most. Taking off too early is also a pitfall, however, because it takes a great deal of board speed to catch the wave.

4. *Paddle for your life.* A common mistake among novice surfers is to stop paddling before they've caught the wave. As a result, they slow down and the wave passes right by them. Very small waves require fast paddling if you're going to get your board speed up and

stay ahead of the wave. Once you feel your board surge, you'll know that you're being propelled by the wave and can stop paddling. If you stop any sooner, though, you run the risk of not catching it at all.

5. *Watch other surfers.* With experience, you'll learn where to line up and when to start paddling. Again, however, you can speed the learning process along by watching other surfers. At first, you'll want to watch from the beach. Keep an eye on the surfers who are consistently catching waves. You'll notice that they tend to always be in the right place at the right time. This is because their experience has taught them how to pick up little signs from the ocean that tell them they need to move in one direction or another. Once you've gained experience of your own, you'll begin to notice more, eventually using it in your own surfing. When you begin to watch other surfers from the lineup, you'll start to pick up on the little things they do to help them catch a wave late or early. If you're respectful and fortunate, you might even get some pointers from the seasoned veterans!

Popping Up

Once you've become proficient at finding the spots to wait for the wave and takeoff, you're ready to start thinking about popping up. The *pop-up* refers to the act of going from a prone or facedown position up onto your feet in one fluid, explosive motion.

1. *Practice first on the beach.* It's best to first practice the pop-up several times on the beach. If you have a difficult time on solid ground, it will be nearly impossible to do it on an unstable, moving surfboard. The first time you attempt it, you'll find that you have a tendency

Pop-Up Tips

1. Practice first on the beach.
2. Arch and look.
3. Keep your hips low and chest up.
4. Focus on consistency.
5. Don't hesitate.

to put one foot in front of the other. Surfers who stand with their left foot forward are called *regular foot.* Those who place their right foot forward are deemed *goofy foot.* The foot you put forward is usually the same as the one you use when you skateboard, snowboard, water-ski, or wakeboard. Surfers who can surf with either foot forward are called *switch foot.* Being switch foot is ideal because it allows you to always surf facing the wave, no matter which way it breaks.

2. *Arch and look.* The first step after you've caught the wave is to lift your chest and stomach off the board so that your back is arched. You can then take a good look toward the peak of the wave to make sure you're not cutting someone off. If you see someone coming, you can stop by dropping your legs into the water and sitting up. It's a lot easier to get out of someone's way *before* you get to your feet.

3. *Keep your hips low and chest up (the "ready position").* Once you're sure you have the right-of-way, you can attempt to pop up. Your feet should be placed shoulder width apart and perpendicular to the board. You'll want to keep your hips low and your chest up. This will help keep your center of gravity low and not too far forward while you attempt to stabilize on a moving surfboard.

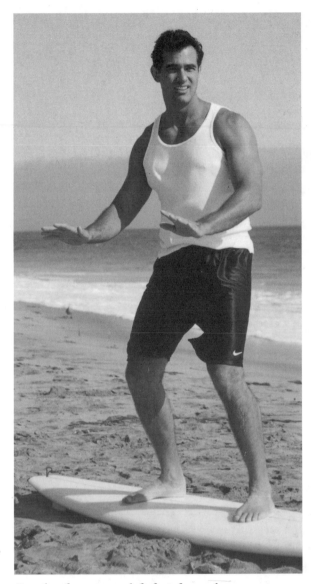

Regular foot-stance, left foot forward.

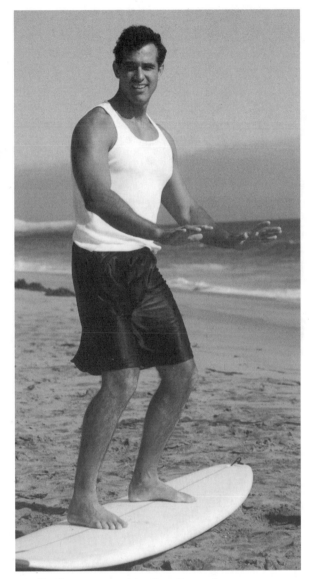

Goofy foot-stance, right foot forward.

4. *Focus on consistency.* When you're first learning, you'll want to focus on consistently placing your feet on the same place on the board. This will allow you to get into a balanced and stable position most quickly. Some people learn to go from their belly to one knee and then stand up. Although this is easier at first, I

find it a difficult habit for people to break as they progress. Being on one knee is a very unstable position and is not very useful at more difficult breaks.

5. *Don't hesitate.* Some breaks require that you pop up immediately after catching the wave, while others can be more forgiving. Either

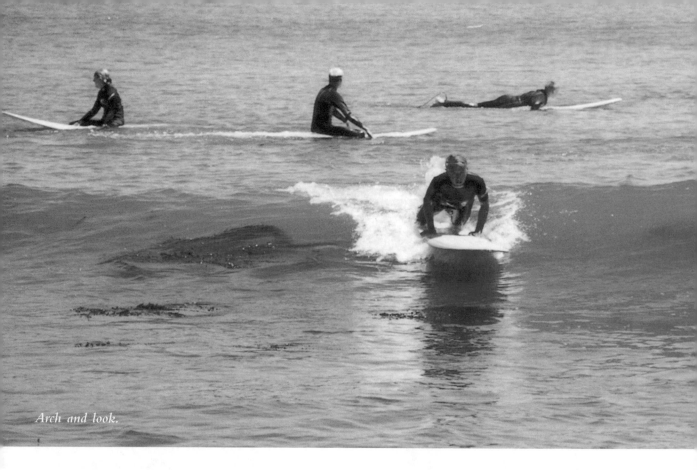

Arch and look.

way, it's important that you learn to pop up without much hesitation. The board is much less stable in whitewater; the longer you wait, the greater the likelihood that you'll be surrounded by it. As you progress, you'll find that the more challenging breaks will require you to get to your feet quickly.

Standing

Once you're consistently popping up you can focus on standing on the board. At first, most beginning surfers tend to assume a survival stance—feet more than shoulder width apart, and upper body bent over at the waist. Try to remember the ready position discussed earlier. If you stand with your feet at shoulder width, your knees bent, and your spine in a neutral position and slightly angled forward, you'll have a much easier time stabilizing.

When you're first learning, it's okay to surf the wave straight toward the beach after you've caught it and popped up. Chances are you'll experience a pretty bumpy ride known as a *roller coaster*, or surfing the whitewater that's created after a wave has broken. As you become more comfortable, however, you'll want to try to surf the face of the wave that hasn't broken yet. This will require a direction change down the line of the wave.

The way you're standing and the type of break you're surfing will affect your ability to make this direction change. If you're standing with your left foot forward (regular foot) and surfing a right (a wave that breaks from left to right), you're surfing *frontside*. If you have your back to the wave, you're surfing *backside*. Standing frontside, or facing the wave while you surf, is easier for most beginners.

Turning

Once you've mastered the pop-up and feel comfortable standing on the board, it's time to focus on turning. Turning a surfboard can be done various ways, depending on the type of board, your speed, and where you are on the wave. When you pressure one rail more than the other, you put the board on edge and it will turn. At slow speeds, turning the board has to be subtler to keep from *digging a rail*—which is when the board starts to sink and come to a stop when it's put on edge. At higher speeds, the board will plane higher in the water, making it possible to execute turns that are much more aggressive and powerful.

When you're beginning, the easiest turn is your toe-side turn. For a regular-footer, it will be easier to turn to the right, and for a goofy-footer, to the left. This means a novice regular foot will have an easier time surfing waves that break from left to right, which allows you to face the wave as you turn and puts you in a more stable position. When you turn on your toe side, you can stay centered more easily because you can make small adjustments at your ankles, knees, and hips while keeping your weight on the balls of your feet. A heel-side turn requires weight farther back on the foot. This makes it more difficult to coordinate for the beginning surfer; you tend to feel like you're falling backward.

When you're starting out, then, think about slightly pressuring the toe-side rail of the board once you've popped up. This is called a *bottom turn*, because you'll be performing it at the bot-

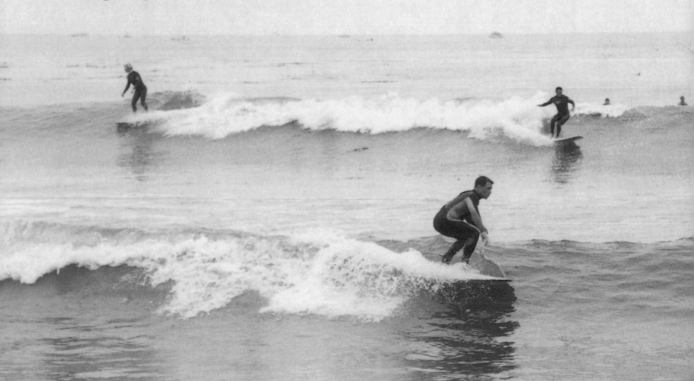

Foreground: Goofy footer surfing frontside.
Back right: Regular footer surfing backside.

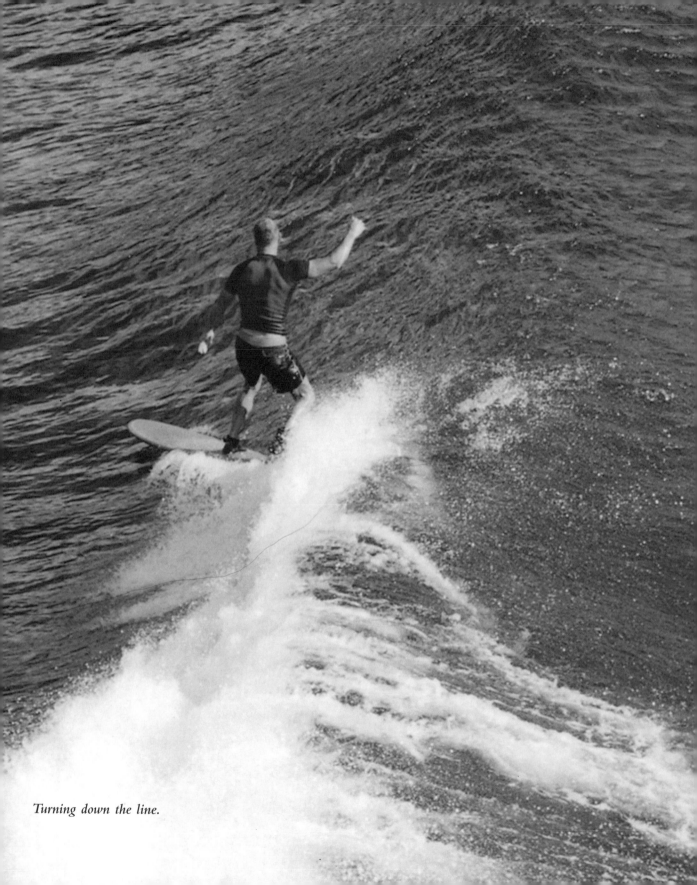

Turning down the line.

tom portion of the wave face. Your goal is to stay where the wave has the most power—in the pocket, just ahead of the breaking part of the wave. If you can keep a longboard in the pocket and in *trim*, or level, you can enjoy nice long rides. After you can perform a bottom turn successfully and on a consistent basis, you can start working on some of the more advanced longboard maneuvers described in chapter 2.

Ending a Ride

At first, the end of your ride will probably be less than graceful. The important thing is that you attempt to hold on to your board. It's best to not get in the habit of jumping off; when it's shallow, this is a good way to sprain your ankle or worse. A novice surfer should strive for a "controlled takedown." In other words, try to gradually sit on your board at the end of a ride. Some beginning surfers get greedy and try to surf a wave all the way to shore. Like drinking, it's important to "know when to say when" if you're surfing a wave close to the beach. Often the wave will close out right before the shore; this will inevitably lead to you and your board becoming separated.

The Inevitable

Falling is simply an aspect of the sport of surfing that every beginner will experience repeatedly. There are numerous terms used to describe the act of losing contact with your surfboard. The most common are *wiping out, taking a header, taking a digger, getting hammered,* and *getting worked.* If you fall as a result of being hit by the breaking lip of the wave, you've been *axed.* One of the more potentially painful and unpleasant moments in surfing is going *over the falls.* This is when you're carried down the wave face by the lip of the wave. It's more apt to happen when the waves are large, and is usually a product of being at the wrong place at the wrong time. Often you'll be driven under water and have the potential of hitting the bottom!

Regardless of what you call your fall, the important thing is that you protect your head and attempt to somehow hold on to your board. Surfers at every level who are challenging themselves should expect to tumble. Still, experienced surfers tend to be able to anticipate falling more quickly and can usually take steps to minimize the impact. As you progress in the sport, your falls will become less frequent and hopefully more graceful!

Be patient with yourself when you're learning to surf, just as with any new skill you're trying to learn. The advanced surfers at your break may make everything look effortless, but they've probably been surfing for years. Try not to get frustrated if you have trouble catching waves or popping up. If you're determined and observant, you'll eventually have the time of your life!

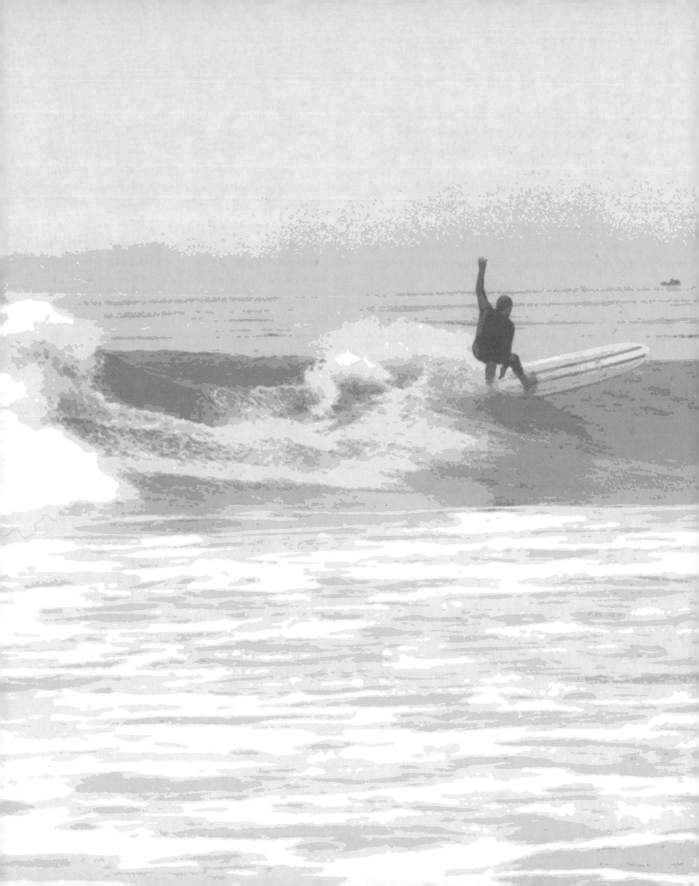

Chapter 2

CLASSIC Advanced Longboarding

To me the best surfer in the world is the person having the most fun. —*Brendan Margieson, professional "free" surfer*

Now that everyone's on the same page, we can get to the good stuff! Try to keep an open mind and think critically about the remaining fourteen chapters. I encourage you to compare your own experience against everything you'll read. And whether or not we're in agreement, I'm confident you'll gain some insight about your surfing.

Before we get to the nuts and bolts of longboarding, let me tell you a bit about how this aspect of the sport has gotten to where it is today.

Throughout much of surfing's history, surfboards were tanks: long, heavy, wide, and made from wood. In the late 1950s, surfboards were still as long as 10 feet, though they were much lighter thanks to fiberglass-and-foam construction. In the late 1960s, shorter, lighter, and more maneuverable boards first became available. This meant more radical maneuvers and tube riding galore. Longboards became "old school." For a while, newcomers to the sport only wanted to ride shortboards. Only the old-timers rode boards more than 8 feet long. In the 1990s, however, surfers began to view longboarding in a different light. Many considered longboarding as *classic*, helping to reignite the sport's popularity.

Shortly thereafter, the surfing world saw numerous design innovations being applied to the average longboard that dramatically improved maneuverability. Today classic longboard designs are still available, but you can also find longboards with newer rocker, rail shape, and bottom characteristics.

In other words, longboarding is cool again!

Advantages

Longboards are clearly the best boards to learn on because they're thicker and more stable. Thickness improves flotation while length aids speed, allowing you to both surf smaller waves and get longer rides.

Longboards can also just be plain fun! Walking around on the board or doing shortboard maneuvers with a high-performance longboard is just another way to experience the sport.

If you're a shortboarder who's grown up believing that longboarding is a waste of time, I urge you to at least give it a try. It will make you a better surfer to have to adapt to different board lengths and shapes. The best surfers I know own both long- and shortboards and will ride whatever the conditions are suited for.

Glide

The term *glide* is used to describe the way a longboard moves through the water. A board that glides well is easier to paddle and catch waves with. Some factors that affect a board's glide include its surface area, thickness, outline, rail shape, rocker, bottom shape, fin shape(s), and the smoothness of its bottom surface. Still, even the nicest gliding board can perform poorly under an inexperienced surfer. Every move that you make on a surfboard will affect its speed and glide, at least to some extent.

Limitations

Longboards can also have their drawbacks. Because of their size, they can be difficult to paddle out through consistent surf. Their flotation is so good that it's tough to submerge them enough to get under an oncoming wave. They also have a much larger *turning radius*—the distance needed to make a direction change—than a shortboard, making them less responsive and requiring more turn setup time.

Advanced Paddling

Because longboards are larger and more stable, they allow more paddling options. For example, some surfers will paddle while sitting, kneeling, or even standing.

Paddling while sitting is fairly easy. Most surfers will put their feet on the side of the board, in order to reduce drag, and pull water with their arms. This isn't the most efficient way to paddle and is generally only used to get into position or to counteract the pull of a slight current.

Paddling while kneeling is a little more difficult and requires greater stability. It does allow different muscles to get involved, however, and can even be used to catch waves. You can stretch your arms out to pull water from a higher angle than lying down. Many surfers also kneel while they're waiting for waves, in an attempt to better see what's behind the incoming swell.

Paddling while standing also requires a fair amount of stability and takes a little practice. This technique is generally used only to generate a tad more board speed after having already caught the wave. The surfer will stand on one leg and use the opposite foot to pull water. Some surfers will also simply crouch down low and use their hands. Either technique does little to increase the board's speed.

Technique

Every movement on the board theoretically has an optimal technique with which it can be performed. Surfing has a long way to go in this area; technique analysis is still a relatively new concept in the sport. Some still argue over which body positions or weight transfers or timing of movements are best, and what is deemed optimal will continue to evolve. Most people, however, will agree that for the most part a particular maneuver is most efficiently performed a certain way. That said, I'm also of the opinion that most of us become set in our perceptions of what's possible and what's ideal. Technique, as with anything else, needs to be thought through critically. The most common way to perform a maneuver might not be the best for you, and thinking "outside the box," or looking at technique from a new perspective, just might lead to a breakthrough for you.

One of the most effective ways to improve your technique is by watching and practicing with surfers who are better than you. This helps you create a mental picture of what you're trying to accomplish. Watching and analyzing video of

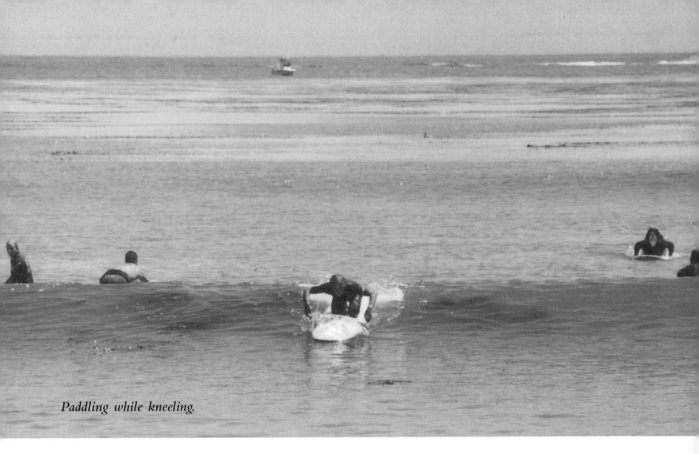

Paddling while kneeling.

yourself and others can also be enormously help-ful. Videos of top pros are sold at most surf shops. And if you have access to a decent cam-corder and a friend, parent, or coach who can film you, you can get some great video footage of yourself surfing. You'll want to find a point or beach break that will allow you to surf within the camera's zoom capabilities. If the image is too far away, you'll obviously lose the ability to analyze the subtleties of your movements. Modern video cameras allow us to slow and pause images frame by frame in order to observe and dissect body positions. In time, video analysis will help you develop the ability to notice the finer points of technique.

For example, take notice of how great long-boarders seem to be able to feel how much of the rail is in contact with the wave during their ride. This knowledge helps them time the initia-tion of their maneuvers as well as knowing how much to pressure one rail or the other. When you watch video of your own surfing, observe things such as how well you link your maneuvers or the fluidity of your movements on the board. Look at the flexion in your ankles, knees, and hips to give you an idea of the point at which you're initiating the most pressure in a turn. Now compare this to video of longboarders you'd like to emulate. Is your upper body "quiet" or are your arms flailing all over the place? As I mentioned before, try to think critically about your surfing—and focus on just one or two things to work on in each session.

There are those in the surfing world who disagree with technique analysis, arguing that it will lead everyone to surf the same. I'm not too concerned that we'll all eventually become clones of each other. Although athletes can learn technique, it's very difficult to adopt someone else's style.

Style

Surfing style is extremely individual and a some-what elusive concept. Unlike technique, style is difficult to analyze because it's essentially an extension of how each surfer connects with the wave. Someone's style might be a combination of how she stands, when she performs certain turns or maneuvers, how fluidly she links movements, or how she seems to flow with the wave. For example, most avid surfers can usually pick out from a distance which one of their friends is riding a wave. This probably isn't because each friend has a radically different technique for each maneuver; instead, it's because each surfer has a slightly different style. From the takeoff to the first turn and on through the entire ride, every surfer has a unique way of putting it all together. And I don't think any of us who surf would want it any other way!

Angling

Once you become comfortable with catching waves, you can attempt *angling*—taking off at an angle to the wave face. When you were first learning, you caught waves by heading directly into shore. This makes it easier to keep the board stable. Angling the board, however, can allow for a later takeoff, because the board is less likely to pearl. It can also eliminate the need for a bottom turn if you angle away from the peak. If you're catching a wave from the shoulder, you might want to angle toward the peak and then make a bottom turn so that you'll be in the pocket of the wave.

Trimming

After you've stood up on a longboard and are following the wave down the line, you can lengthen your ride by keeping the board in trim.

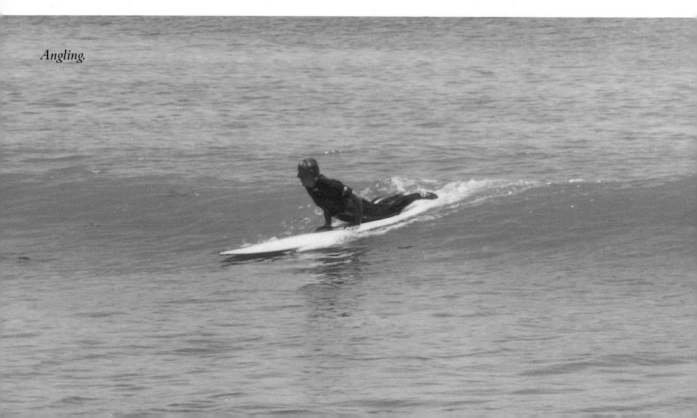

Angling.

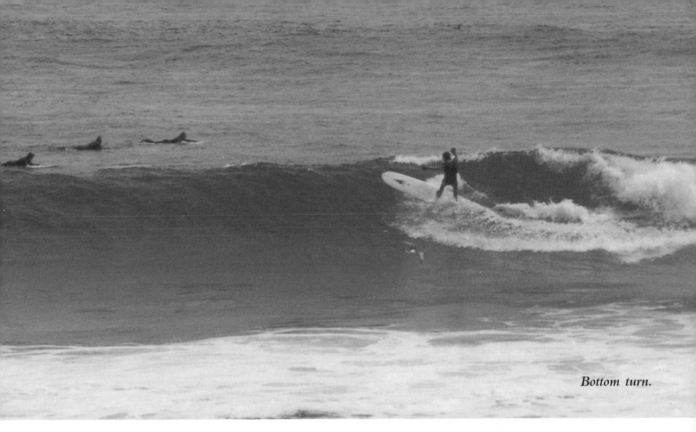

Bottom turn.

Trimming is the act of adjusting your weight on a surfboard both fore and aft and laterally in order to keep it level, thus maximizing board speed. Advanced longboarders can quickly make these adjustments by walking back and forth on the board. As they move forward, the board will speed up as it tracks down the face of the wave. As they move backward, the board slows down as the tail starts to push more water.

The ability to manage your speed will give you maximum control and will allow you to "work" the wave all the way to the beach. If you watch very experienced longboarders, you'll notice that they use a combination of turns and trimming adjustments to stay in the pocket of the wave where they can develop speed.

Setting Up

Because longboards have a longer turning radius, it's sometimes necessary to set up. This simply entails getting the board into an ideal position

on the wave in order to perform a maneuver such as turning. There are times when you might want to stall the board or slow it down. For example, if you've gained too much speed and find yourself surfing slightly ahead of the wave, you might want to adjust your weight back on the board. This will slow the board down and perhaps get you back into the pocket. Many find this to be an easy way to reposition the board on the wave without changing direction.

Turning

The basic longboarding turns are the bottom turn, top turn, and cut back . . . and you can't truly surf a longboard without knowing how to do all three!

Bottom-Turn Technique

A *bottom turn* consists of turning the board at the bottom of the wave face. For instance, if you're on a wave that's breaking right, you might want to perform a bottom turn to the right immediately after taking off on the wave. If you'd taken off at the peak of the wave, this would more than likely put you in the pocket.

1. Carry your speed from the pocket of the wave to the bottom of the wave face.
2. From the middle of the board, keep your hips and shoulders level and your hands forward.
3. As the board is put on edge, bend your knees and ankles and push them forward into the turn.
4. At the apex of the turn, your upper body is angled toward the wave and the inside rail is evenly weighted.
5. As you complete the turn, keep your ankles and knees soft to allow the board to return under your body.

Top-Turn Technique

A *top turn* is one in which you turn the board from high on the wave face toward the bottom. This is usually done in order to generate more speed and is often linked with a bottom turn. It's common to see advanced surfers alternating top and bottom turns all the way down a wave's face.

1. Carry your speed from the pocket of the wave to the top portion of the wave face.
2. Stand in the middle or rear of the board with level hips and chest up as you initiate the turn.
3. Push your weight through your back foot and the rear, inside rail while keeping your upper body forward.
4. Rotate your upper body slightly toward the pit as the board begins to accelerate through the arc.
5. At the end of the turn, center your weight with your hips low and upper body forward.

Cut-Back Technique

A *cut back* is a turn usually performed on the shoulder toward the breaking part of the wave. For example, if you're on a wave that's breaking left, you might want to perform a cut back to the right in order to get back to where the wave has more power.

1. Carry your speed from the wave face onto the wave shoulder.
2. Stand toward the rear of the board with level hips and shoulders as you put the board on edge.
3. Rotate your upper body slightly and roll your knees and ankles forward into the turn.
4. Keep your weight over the back half of the inside rail through the arc of the turn.
5. Keep your hips low, chest up, and upper body forward as you complete the turn and the board levels out.

It's common to see longboarders link cut back and bottom turns. They might use a cut back to get back into the pocket and then without delay move into a bottom turn to follow the

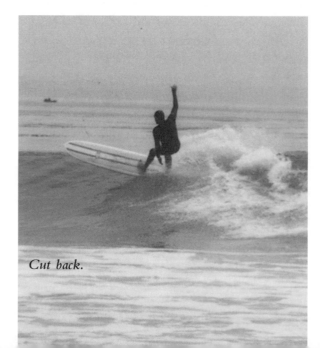

Cut back.

direction of the breaking wave. The goal is to execute both turns as fluidly as possible in order to maintain board speed.

Bottom turns, top turns, and cut backs can be performed while you're standing in either the middle or rear portion of the board. Moving to the rear of the board will free the rails and cause the board to stall slightly, but it also allows the direction change to be made more quickly. Often, advanced longboarders will move to the rear of the board in order to make a sweeping arc; then they'll immediately walk forward again in order to trim the board. If the wave is small and relatively slow, you might want to make a more subtle direction change so as to not lose as much momentum. How each turn is performed will depend on numerous factors, including the shape of the wave, the speed of the board, the next maneuver desired, and your own abilities.

The *kick out* is one way advanced surfers end a ride by turning out of a wave. It's most commonly used in order to avoid getting hammered by a wave that's closing out or to avoid another surfer who has the right-of-way on a wave. As with most other turns, you place more weight on the rear of the surfboard in order to free the rails and swing the board over the lip. Once the board is over the lip, you can drop down to a paddling position. Now you're poised to get back out to the line-up.

Walking the Nose

Walking up and back on a moving surfboard requires a great deal of stability, wave knowledge, and timing. An advanced longboarder has developed a sense for when it's time to move forward or back on the board in order to keep it in trim, stay in the pocket, adjust speed, or perform a maneuver.

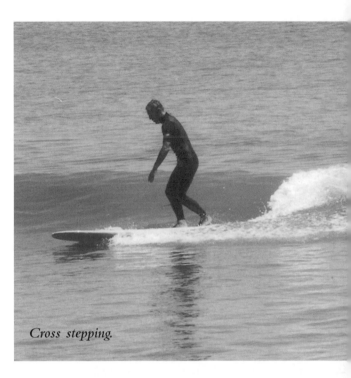

Cross stepping.

At first, novice longboarders will shuffle their feet up and back on the board in an attempt to adjust their weight. This approach is effective but awkward and relatively slow. The preferred method of walking on a moving surfboard, called *cross stepping,* simply involves placing one foot laterally in front of the other to move forward or back on a longboard. The key is sensing when to begin stepping, how quickly to step, how big a step to take, and how much weight to place on each foot while you're stepping. Your footwork will ultimately depend on the board's steadiness, which is influenced by factors such as your weight and stability, board speed, and wave shape. When done well, cross stepping makes walking on a longboard look very fluid and graceful.

Cross stepping gives a longboarder an opportunity to master the art of *nose riding.* Many have described surfing on the front section of a longboard to be one of the sport's greatest thrills. To not see your board while riding a wave gives the illusion of hovering above the water and can border on addiction! Before you can move forward on the board, however, it's important to first set the inside rail, or the rail turning into the wave. Once that side of the surfboard is stable, it also helps if the tail of the board is held down by the breaking part of the wave. When both the inside rail and tail are secure at the same time, you've created a nice, steady platform on which to dance!

Hanging five is an advanced longboarding maneuver in which one foot—five toes—is placed on the very nose of the board. The other foot may be well behind the front foot, and often surfers will drop their hips in order to increase stability.

Hanging ten is a very advanced longboarding maneuver in which both feet, or ten toes, are placed on the very nose of the board. The amount of time you spend up there will depend on how the board and wave are reacting to one another. The longest nose rides can be experienced on medium-size and fast-developing waves. Once you've generated a decent amount of speed and have anchored the tail of the board in the curl, you can stand on the nose until the wave slows down or closes out. But if you stand up there too long, the tail of the board will break free and flip up into the air. Most advanced longboarders will step back toward the tail or simply sit down on the board as soon as they sense the slightest instability. Veteran longboarders can squeeze every possible second out of a nose ride without overstaying their welcome!

Other Advanced Maneuvers

There are numerous things you can do on a longboard. As you progress, you'll begin to push the edge of the envelope of possibilities. Board shape, wave shape, speed, physics, athleticism, and creativity are your only limitations! What follows are a few examples of the more advanced longboarding maneuvers.

- *Reentry.* This is an advanced maneuver performed off the lip of a breaking wave. It's essentially an aggressive top turn in which the board is turned from the lip toward the pit of the wave.
- *Floater.* Another advanced maneuver in which the board is actually launched off the lip and you land in the whitewater. Floaters are most commonly executed when you realize that a wave will close out ahead of you. Sometimes you may be able to ride around the section that has closed out to find smooth water again. In other cases your ride could be extended if the wave reforms after you've performed a floater.
- **Getting tubed, barreled, or shacked.** This is one of the greatest feelings in the sport of surfing. It involves being completely covered by the falling lip. Shallow reef breaks are famous for providing some of the world's best barrel rides. The bigger the wave, the more upright you can stand in the tube. Getting barreled on a longboard takes a great deal of skill. Taking off on a tubing wave requires aggressive angling; also, because a longer board is generally less responsive, getting into position for a tube ride can be difficult. If you're fortunate enough to pull it off, however, you will know the true meaning of the word *stoked*.
- *Switch-foot hop.* In this fun little maneuver, you jump vertically off your board, rotate 180 degrees in the air, and land back on the board facing the opposite direction. The challenge is to take off and land softly so as to not cause the board to dig a rail. If you can surf with either foot forward, the switch-foot hop allows

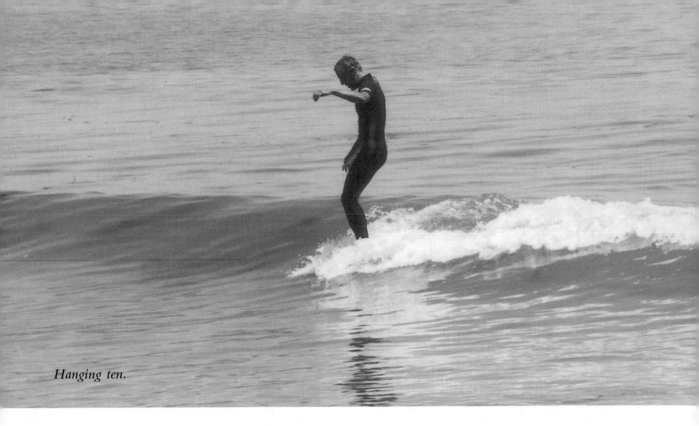

Hanging ten.

you to make direction changes and still surf a wave either frontside or backside. Learning how to pop up with either foot forward is also incredibly helpful in facing the wave while you surf.

- *Helicopter or nose 360.* A very advanced maneuver in which you spin the board 360 degrees while you stand on the nose. Because all of your weight is on the front part of the board, the rails and fins are free to move laterally. Helicopters require very quick feet and a great deal of practice!

- *Headstand.* Like the helicopter, the headstand, or surfing upside down, requires a fair amount of trial and error. Clearly, if your headstands on the beach are wobbly, you'll have virtually no chance of executing one on a moving surfboard. Once you've perfected the maneuver on dry land, the challenge is to be able to stabilize the board as you bring your legs to the vertical position.

- *Aerials.* Some advanced longboarders on

high-performance boards are even pulling off aerials. An aerial maneuver entails getting air on a surfboard by launching it off the lip of the wave. This takes a lot of speed and very good timing if you're to move that much board into the air.

Now get out there and invent some maneuvers of your own!

Final Note

You'll probably see a lot of experienced long-boarders performing the above maneuvers without a leash. This is, hopefully, because they have excellent control over their boards and are extremely confident that they won't be placing anyone else in danger. Unfortunately, no matter what your skill level, factors such as other surfers, kelp, and wave action aren't always under your control. As a result, I recommend that you always use a leash while surfing. And please don't attempt any of the moves described in this book until you're certain that your actions aren't placing others at risk.

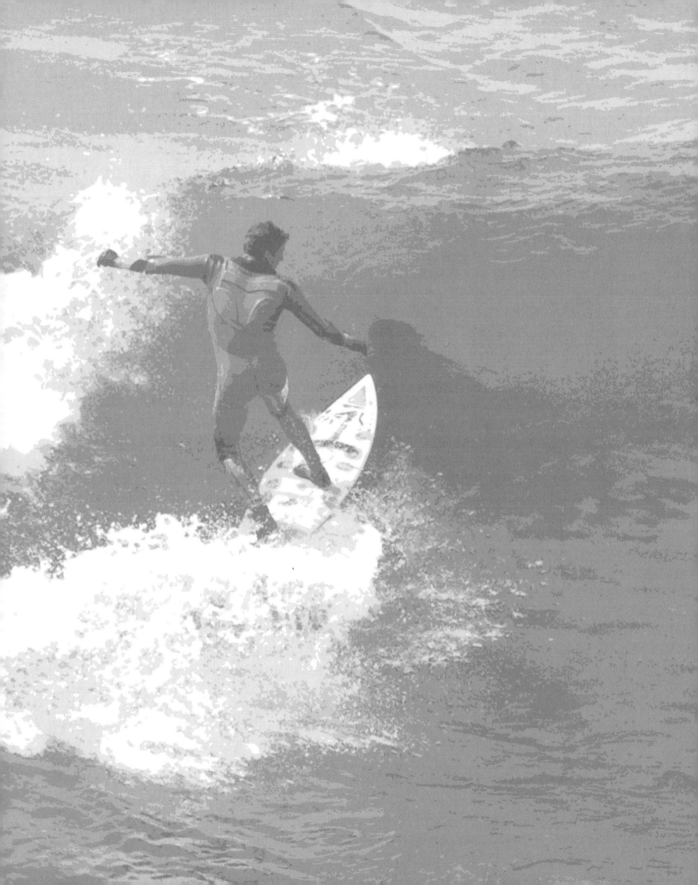

Chapter 3

SLASH Shortboarding

Surfing's come a long way and it's got a long way to go. —*Sunny Garcia, professional surfer, 2000 world champion*

As surfing became more and more popular, shapers started to experiment with different materials, shapes, and lengths. The advent of fiberglass-and-foam boards and new fin configurations accelerated design innovations further. Eventually shapers created what we now refer to as shortboards. The modern shortboard has taken a variety of shapes, lengths, and fin configurations. For the most part, shortboards are designed to be light and highly maneuverable. They are usually less than 7 feet and have an oblong shape with significant rocker at the nose and tail.

Old School versus New School

Most people these days associate surfing with shortboarding. Although longboard design and maneuverability are continually evolving, many younger surfers still view longboarding as being "old school" or dated. In fact, both styles of surfing and types of boards can be considered "new school," depending on your perspective. Go to any break and you'll see surfers pushing the limits with all sizes and shapes of boards. Most accomplished surfers recognize the value of all types and styles of surfing and have a variety of boards in their quiver. Personally, I choose my equipment according to my mood and the surf conditions. I urge you to do the same!

Advantages

The main reason many advanced surfers ride shortboards is their responsiveness. A shorter board can be turned with the slightest amount of weight transfer. Their shape and length make shortboards much easier to put on edge and change direction in a very short turning radius or *arc*—a term used to describe the path of a turning board.

Shortboards also allow you to catch a wave later than on a longer board. Because the tail of a shortboard isn't picked up as much by the approaching wave, you can catch a breaking wave more easily. The narrow nose and rocker helps keep the front of the board from submerging on a late takeoff.

Shortboards are also preferable when taking off on hollow waves with very steep faces. It's common to get some air when taking off on such a wave. This is called a *drop*: surfer and board becoming airborne when entering steep or large waves.

A shorter board will meet the wave face sooner than a larger board, which tends to float a

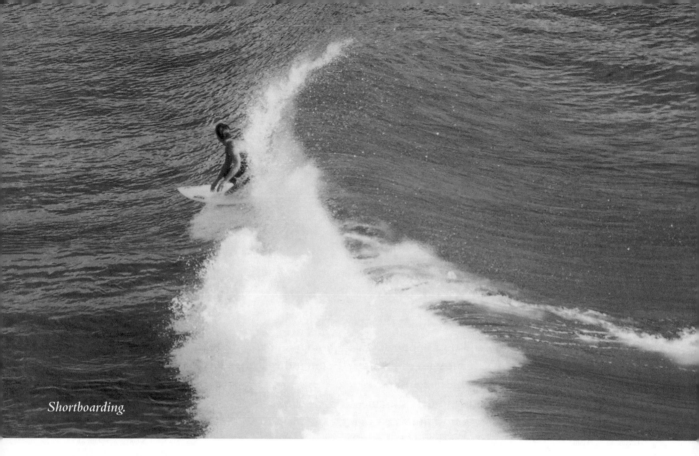

Shortboarding.

little longer. As a result, a shortboard will increase your chance of making the drop successfully.

Additionally, shortboards make it much easier to paddle out to the lineup on a big day. You can duck-dive and get under a breaking wave more easily because shortboards are less buoyant.

Maneuverability

The difference in responsiveness between a shortboard and longboard is analogous to the differences between a Porsche and a Suburban. At 40 miles per hour, a Porsche can corner precisely and instantaneously on a mountain road. At the same speed, a Suburban would need much more room and time to negotiate the corner. Similarly, a shortboard requires very little setup and can be virtually willed into a tight-radius turn.

Limitations

Because shortboards are thinner, shorter, and have more rocker than longboards, they require more energy to paddle. As a result, it is more difficult to catch small waves or to catch waves early with a smaller board. The smaller surface area of a shortboard translates to little or no glide. Thus, it's common to see shortboarders *pumping the board,* or pushing it up and down a wave face in an effort to generate more speed.

Shorter boards are also less stable for the novice surfer. A beginner will find it much more difficult to paddle, sit, pop up, stand or turn on a shortboard. The characteristics of most shortboards make them more "squirrelly" and more difficult to stay centered on than a longboard.

Heavier surfers will also have a more difficult time with shorter boards. A thin shortboard has very little buoyancy and will sink easily at slow speeds when ridden by larger surfers. As a result, many bigger surfers have a shaper design a slightly thicker, wider, and longer board that will still handle like a shortboard under their weight.

Technique

As noted in chapter 2, every movement on the board theoretically has an optimal technique with which it can be performed. Because technique analysis is still relatively new in the sport, shortboard surfing, like longboard surfing, has a long way to go in this area—but there's a great deal to be learned from this practice.

Video analysis has been an integral part of training in other skill sports, such as ski racing, for decades. Numerous subtleties—weight transfers, body positions, timing—are very difficult to see in real time. Video allows a surfer and coach to look at movement one frame at a time in order to identify areas to work on. At the competition level, I urge surfers to watch video of themselves as well as of top pros to give them a mental picture of how a particular maneuver or turn could be better executed. After a while, most athletes develop a better understanding of surf technique, which directly results in improvements.

As we discussed in chapter 2, think critically about your surfing. Check out the videos of pro surfers at your local surf shop and borrow or buy an affordable or even used video camera to get some film of yourself. You don't need anything too fancy. Any camcorder that will provide a decent image of a moving object 50 to 100 yards from the beach will work. Have a friend, parent, or coach film you for thirty or forty minutes at a break that's relatively close to shore. When you watch video of yourself and others, try to notice the timing and amount of pressure put on the rail

during a turn. Initiation of pressure can make a big difference in turn shape. Are you trying to make a full, sweeping arc or attempting to take a chunk out of the lip? Compare the flexion of your ankles, knees, and hips in various stages of the turn with that of surfers whom you think are better than you. Take notice of upper-body movements, hand positions, and where a surfer is looking during a maneuver. The more you analyze technique, the less you'll feel you know. This is healthy, for it will keep you striving for more knowledge and better refinement of your surfing.

Style

As I mentioned earlier, although athletes can learn technique, it is very difficult to adopt the style of others. Shortboarding style is difficult to analyze because, as with longboarding, it's very individualistic and essentially an extension of how a surfer connects with the wave. Style is a combination of so many things. For example, two surfers might have virtually identical techniques for performing a bottom turn, but when you take into consideration their timing, fluidity, power, stance, the way they link turns, and the type of maneuvers they perform, you will probably conclude that they have different styles. Surfers' styles are created through years of surfing and are influenced by factors such as their body types, where they've surfed, the type of equipment they've used, and the level of surfing they've been exposed to. A lot of emphasis has been placed on this subject over the years because the ability to develop a unique style can truly separate the good from the great.

Speed

The key to improving your performance and having more fun is to find ways to generate speed. The quality of your turns, maneuvers, and aerials are all speed-dependent. And, in general, the biggest difference between the pros and the average surfer is the velocity at which the pros are traveling. Most surfers are moving too slowly to execute a ballistic cut back or boost a radical air! On the other hand, once you've created speed, you need to know how to manage it so you can "work" the wave optimally. The act of turning can help you either generate or dump speed. It all hinges on where you perform the turn, when you start the turn, and the shape and speed of the wave. For example, a cut back on the shoulder of the wave will help you bleed off some speed in order to get back in the pocket so you can accelerate again. And, a series of top and bottom turns down the wave face can help you reach the velocity necessary for a sick aerial! Spend time watching how the best surfers at your break create and use speed, and then try to incorporate it into your own surfing.

Turning

As I've mentioned, most shortboards are designed to excel once they're put on edge. Advanced shortboarders can draw powerful and fluid lines in a wave when they surf. The very best make direction changes look effortless: Every turn is linked and seems to flow with the contours of the wave.

When I first began coaching shortboarders, the emphasis was on drawing and linking powerful arcs in the wave. Sliding the tail around was a big no-no. Now there are some maneuvers in which you intentionally try to break the tail or the nose of the board free. Still, the foundation of all great surfing is knowing the subtle intricacies of completely committing to a surfboard's rail and executing full, sweeping arcs. In other

words, all shortboard maneuvers start with the ability to carve any type of turn at will. As with any sport, keep in mind that there's a progression in surfing. Just as a child learns to crawl before he walks and walks before he runs, the path to radical off-the-lip maneuvers and big air begins with performing the following turns flawlessly.

As in longboarding, the basic shortboarding turns are the *bottom turn, top turn,* and *cut back.* But unlike longboarding—where you move up and back—on a shortboard your feet are almost always in the same place on the board.

Bottom-Turn Technique

A bottom turn consists of turning the board at the bottom of the wave face. This turn is used frequently to gain speed, set up a maneuver, and get to the pocket or to get barreled.

1. Carry your speed from the wave face to the pit of the wave.
2. Anticipate the amount of arc required to complete the turn, get into position, and conserve your speed.
3. As you put the board on edge, keep your knees bent, hips and shoulders level, and hands forward.
4. At the apex of the turn, the upper body is angled toward the wave and the inside rail is evenly and fully weighted.
5. At the end of the turn, soft ankles and knees allow the board to return under your weight.

Top-Turn Technique

In a top turn, the board is turned from high on the wave face toward the bottom. This is usually done in order to generate more speed and often linked with another turn or maneuver.

1. Carry your speed from the pocket of the wave toward the lip.

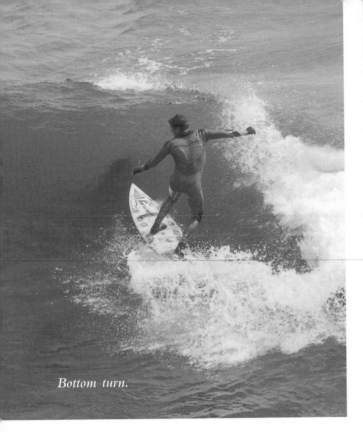

Bottom turn.

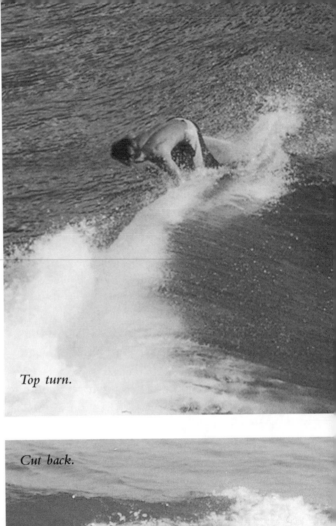

Top turn.

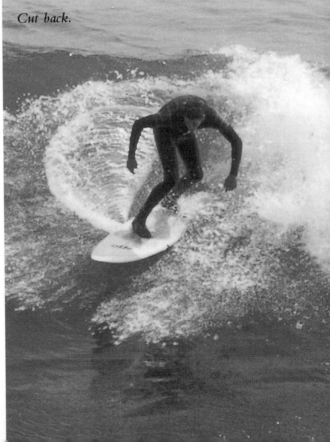

Cut back.

2. Focus on the turn's completion point based on the wave shape and your evaluation of how it's breaking.
3. At the initiation of the turn, keep your hips low, with your shoulders and hips level and rotated toward the bottom of the wave.
4. At the apex of the turn, your weight is on the back half of the inside rail. Pull the board around by rotating your upper body.
5. At the completion of the turn, keep your chest up and your knees and ankles flexed with your weight centered and the board level.

Cut-Back Technique

A cut back turn is typically performed on the shoulder toward the peak of the wave. Cut backs generally have a greater arc than do bottom or top turns. As a result of this more radical direction change and the fact that the point is usually to move laterally on the wave, not vertically, cut backs often result in a loss of speed. Still, entering the turn with more momentum and properly timing your entrance to the pocket of the wave can quickly lead to acceleration of the board once again.

1. Carry your speed from the wave face onto the wave shoulder.
2. Maintain level hips and shoulders and a relatively quiet upper body as you put the board on edge.
3. Rotate your upper body slightly, hands forward, and roll your knees and ankles into the turn.
4. Keep your weight over the back half of the inside rail and your chest up through the arc of the turn.
5. Keep your hips low, your weight centered, and your upper body forward as you finish the turn and the board levels out.

As with longboarding, the goal in turning a shortboard is generally to execute and link arcs as fluidly as possible in order to maintain board speed. When you fully commit to the inside rail and submerge the edge of the board in an aggressive and powerful arc, you should be prepared to lose a significant amount of board speed. If you time the release of the pressure from the rail at the right moment and with the right body position, however, the board will accelerate. Some surfers and photographers like those turns that result in a huge spray of water shooting out from the bottom of the board. For the average surfers, though, this may mean losing so much momentum that they lose their position in the pocket and are unable to set up for any other turns or maneuvers. It's all about trade-offs.

There are also variations on the three basic turns described above. For example, a more subtle direction change called a fade might be used to set up for another turn or maneuver. Which turn is used and how it's executed will depend on factors that can include wave shape, board speed, the next maneuver desired, and your own abilities.

Maneuvers

There are quite possibly hundreds of shortboarding maneuvers being performed worldwide today. Maneuvers usually start as a turn and differ from one another in such factors as where the board is positioned on the wave, the surfer's stance, the surfer's body position, the arc of the turn, or what's done in the air.

For instance, a top turn that is performed with your back to the wave and where you drive the board against the lip is called a backside top turn/lip bounce. There are also variations on the cut back. There's the short arc roundhouse cut back, semi-layback cut back, and full rail cut back.

Fortunately, the names of most maneuvers generally resemble their appearance. Still, some maneuvers have multiple or obscure names that can make things more complicated.

What follows are a few of the most commonly executed shortboarding maneuvers.

Floater Reentry Technique

A *reentry* is an advanced maneuver performed off the lip of a breaking wave. It's essentially an aggressive top turn in which the board is turned from the lip toward the pit of the wave. Other examples include the tailslide reentry, foam bounce reentry, and floater reentry.

A *floater* is also an advanced maneuver in which the board is actually launched off the lip and the surfer lands in the whitewater. Variations on this one include the tweaked floater, with-the-lip floater, and floater reentry. Of these, the latter is one of the more commonly performed. Here you turn onto and then "float" down with the falling lip.

1. Anticipate and set up as wave is breaking in front of you down the line.
2. Carry your speed off the wave face with your chest up, knees bent, hips low, and hands forward.
3. Launch the board off the lip, keeping your compact position and angling slightly toward the shore.
4. While in the air, look for your landing, keeping your knees bent and hips, shoulders, and board level.
5. Your hips, knees, and ankles should be soft and slightly flexed to gradually absorb the landing.

Snap Technique

Another common advanced shortboarding maneuver, the snap involves making a 180-degree turn vertically on the wave face. Variations on the snap include the backside vertical snap, tailslide snap, and layback snap.

1. Carry a lot of speed through a bottom turn up the wave face.
2. Keep your shoulders and hips level, your hands forward, your knees bent, and your chest up.
3. Push your weight through your back foot and the rear inside rail while keeping your upper body forward.
4. As the board accelerates vertically, rotate your upper body toward the pit while keeping your weight on your back foot.
5. At the finish of the turn, your weight should be centered, with your hips low and your upper body forward.

Tube Ride Technique

As I mentioned in chapter 2, getting tubed is one

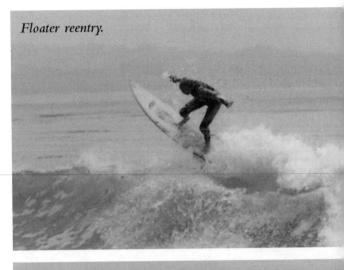

Floater reentry.

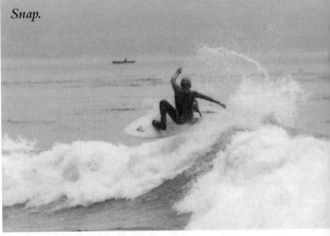

Snap.

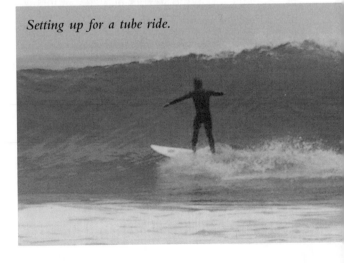

Setting up for a tube ride.

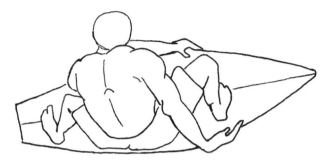

Double grab air

Both hands are on the rails.

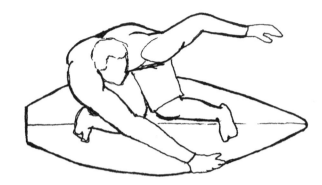

Indy grab air

Your back hand is on the toe-side rail.

of the greatest feelings in the sport of surfing. It involves being completely covered by the falling lip. Shallow reef breaks are famous for providing some of the world's best barrel rides. The bigger the wave, the more upright you can stand in the tube. The *deeper* the tube ride, or farther back in the tube you are, the more difficult it is to exit before the wave closes out. If you're very deep during a tube ride, you might be racing toward a very narrow opening in the wave. Larger waves can *spit*, or force spraying water out of the barrel toward you as the tube collapses. This can make it very difficult for you to see but provides an intense rush! Different versions of the tube ride consist of the rail-grab tube ride and backside tube ride.

1. First, set up and time a turn that allows pulling the board under the breaking part of the wave.
2. Control your board speed to stay deep enough to be covered, but not so deep that you can't exit.
3. Set the inside rail into the wave face while keeping your weight, ankles, and knees forward and the board in trim.
4. Keep your hips low and your upper body

relaxed, making subtle board and body adjustments inside the tube.
5. Stall the board to lengthen the ride and push your weight forward to exit. Once you're out, celebrate!

Grab-Air Technique

Getting air, or launching off the lip, on a surfboard has led to some of the more advanced maneuvers being performed. Many shapers have boards available that are specifically designed for getting air. There are numerous types of airs and in some instances multiple names for the same maneuvers. Aerial maneuvers are generally differentiated by whether the rider holds the board in the air or not—grab air and no-grab-air, respectively. Airs also differ according to the amount of rotation performed in the air and where the board is held while in flight. For instance, a 360 no-grab-air involves one complete rotation, while in a roast beef grab your rear hand grabs the heel rail between your legs.

1. Look for a steep, smooth section of the wave face at the lip that can serve as a launching point.

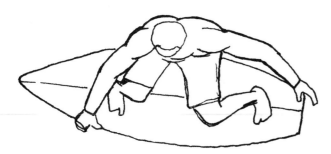

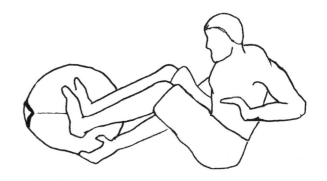

Mute grab air

Your front hand is on the toe-side rail.

Stalefish grab air

Your back hand is on the heel-side rail.

2. Generate and carry a lot of speed in order to angle the board up the wave face and beyond.
3. Hold a compact body position with level shoulders, extending your arms up and forward at the launch point.
4. While in the air, grab the board to keep in contact with it and at the same time look for a good landing.
5. Upon descent, release your grab on the board while keeping your weight forward and your knees flexed to absorb the landing.

The Future

As I noted in chapter 1, the incorporation of flex in surfboard design is sure to revolutionize the sport. Dual-directional boards are also being experimented with and could open up a whole new range of possible maneuvers. Yet what seems most promising of all is that every year we are seeing more aggressive, powerful, and creative surfing as athletes become better conditioned, more skillful, more knowledgeable, and hence better able to take advantage of equipment advances. The future of advanced shortboard surfing indeed looks very bright!

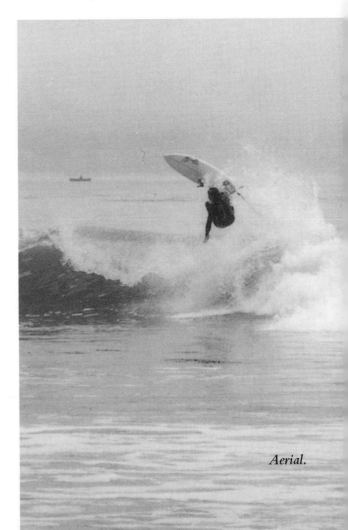

Aerial.

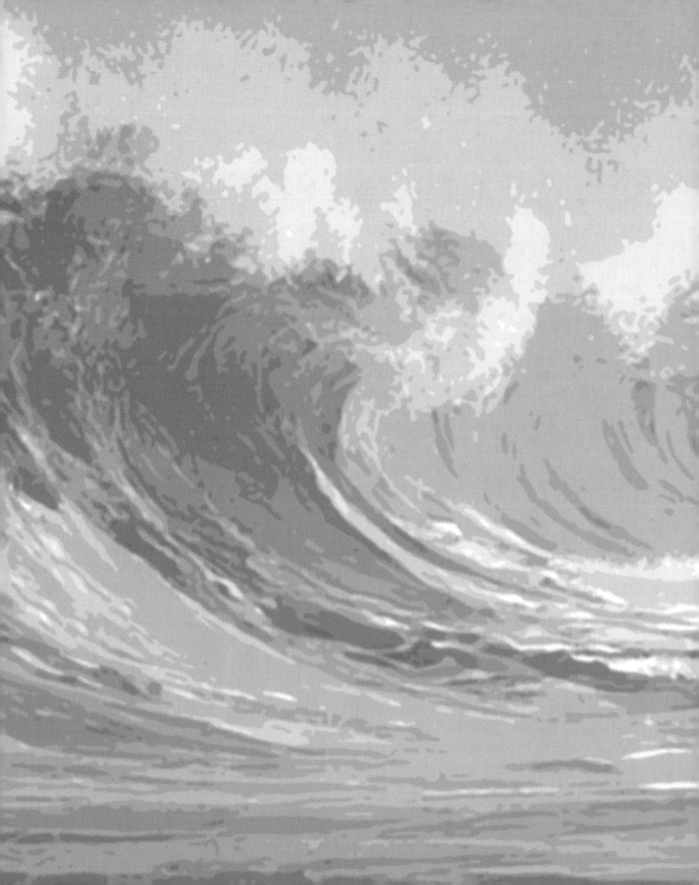

Chapter 4

MONSTERS Big-Wave Surfing

The only way you can really prepare for big waves is to ride big waves. And we'll go out there and do it . . . maybe we'll die trying, but we'll go out and give it a shot. I'm not afraid of dying like that. To me it's not tragic to die doing something you love. —*Mark Foo, a well-known big-wave surfer who drowned at Maverick's, Half Moon Bay, California, while surfing big waves in 1994*

Big-wave surfing—surfing waves with faces more than 20 feet high—has received a great deal of attention in the last ten years. And understandably so, because enormous waves are one of the most powerful and intriguing forces of nature. Surfers and nonsurfers alike can almost feel the adrenaline rush of big-wave surfing simply by looking at photos and video footage of surfers being dwarfed by 40-, 50-, 60-, even 70-foot walls of water.

Genuine big waves occur only in certain parts of the world. This is because it takes a special set of circumstances to create this kind of surf. Big waves obviously require a well-organized swell with a tremendous amount of energy. Such a swell is usually created in the open ocean by very large winter storms. Each hemisphere might experience a storm with this kind of energy potential perhaps ten to twenty times a year. Often the big-wave swell then has to travel thousands of miles, through very deep water, before reaching an area of shallower water where it can form a wave. It's possible that other swell

energy and wind energy focused in the opposite direction could dissipate a potential big-wave swell before it reaches any relatively shallow water. To complicate matters further, it's also possible that the large swell could lose a great deal of energy if it encounters an open-ocean reef or shelf before it arrives at a deep-water break that surfers can access. As a result, the best big-wave spots in the world are lucky to get more than thirty days of waves over 15 feet each winter.

And yet, when everything comes together just right, surfers are treated to a large, powerful, and magical show of nature's force!

The Big-Wave Subculture

Big-wave surfers, or *hellmen* and *hellwomen,* are a subculture within the subculture of surfing. What has historically separated big-wave surfers from the rest of society is that they voluntarily subject themselves to extreme danger without much external motivation. Most men and women who ride truly large waves (20-plus feet) do so with little recognition or money as a reward. Big-wave

Big-Wave Timeline

1917
Duke Kahanamoku rides a very large wave on the South Shore of Oahu in one of the earliest "big-wave" surfing attempts reported.

1943
Dickie Cross drowns attempting to paddle in on a big day in Waimea Bay. As one of the best-known and most respected surfers and watermen of his day, Dickie's death convinces many that big-wave surfing is not worth the risk.

1953
Buzzy Trent, George Downing, and Wally Froiseth ride what is reported as a wave over 20 feet, at Makaha in Hawaii.

1964
Greg Noll rides a wave that is reportedly even larger than the one surfed in 1953, at Outside Pipeline in Hawaii.

1975
Jeff Clark surfs Maverick's, located in Half Moon Bay, California, for the first time. Maverick's is today regarded as one of the most challenging big-wave surf spots in the world.

1988
Darrick Doerner catches a wave taller than 40 feet at Waimea Bay—considered one of the biggest ever ridden.

1991
Laird Hamilton and Buzzy Kerbox tow into a wave well over 40 feet at Phantom's.

1994
Hawaiian big-wave surfer Mark Foo dies while surfing at Maverick's. It's the first time he has surfed this break.

1998
Ken Bradshaw is towed into one of the biggest waves ever ridden, on the Hawaiian island of Oahu. Some accounts estimate the wave as having a face nearly five stories high.

1999
Noah Johnson wins $55,000 at the Quiksilver Invitational in 20-foot Waimea Bay. This marks the first time a significant amount of money is offered at a big-wave contest.

2001
Mike Parsons tows into a 66-footer at Cortes Bank and wins $60,000 from swell.com. This is the biggest wave ever surfed, as well as the most amount of money awarded to a big-wave surfer.

2002
Garrett McNamara and Rodrigo Resende win $70,000 at the Tow-in World Cup at Jaws, again upping the ante for big-wave surfing prize money.

riders are a different breed and comprise far less than 1 percent of all surfers.

Big-wave surfing has its own lifestyle, too. Many of these surfers live on the North Shore of the Hawaiian island of Oahu—considered the mecca of the sport with some of the world's most consistent big-wave surf. Surfers who want to focus on big-wave riding and immerse themselves in the lifestyle flock there. These "diehards" will occasionally travel to other spots in the world when they hear that the surf is expected to be bigger than what's at home. The most accomplished seem unconcerned with the competitive and image aspects that preoccupy the rest of the sport. They're very independent athletes driven by their next big-wave experience. They all have a tremendous amount of knowledge and respect for the ocean but are also eager to push the limits of what's possible—and as a result challenge death.

The sport of big-wave surfing takes a great deal of skill and preparation. These surfers are true watermen and waterwomen. Surfing big waves requires a considerable amount of physical conditioning and athleticism. Often these large waves are so far from shore that, surfing them, you can barely see land. Some break miles into the open ocean.

These are intense, focused individuals. Everything they do revolves around their ability to ride big waves. They are motivated by the prospect of new and greater challenges. Obviously, a high level of adrenaline and fear accompanies being in the ocean at its most unpredictable and powerful. The subculture of big-wave surfing can perhaps best be described as *unique*. Many would call these men and women eccentric or even crazy. Others view them as great athletes who share common characteristics that enable them to accomplish amaz-

ing, death-defying feats. Either way, you have to envy their passion for what they do and their ability to lead a lifestyle that allows them to pursue what they love.

Locations

Here are the best-known and most respected spots where you can find huge surf a few times each year:

- *Cortes Bank,* 100 miles off the coast of San Diego, California.
- *Easter Reef,* Southern Australia.
- *Jaws,* Maui, Hawaii.
- *Killers,* Todos Santos, Mexico.
- *King's Reef,* an outer reef in Hawaii.
- *Makaha,* Oahu, Hawaii.
- *Margaret River,* Southern Australia.
- *Maverick's,* Half Moon Bay, California.
- *Outside Log Cabins,* Oahu, Hawaii.
- *Waimea Bay,* Oahu, Hawaii.

There are other ominous spots around, too:

- *Backdoor,* Oahu, Hawaii.
- *Desert Point,* Lombok, Indonesia.
- *Pipeline,* Oahu, Hawaii.
- *Puerto Escondido,* Mexico.
- *Shark Island,* Australia.
- *Teahupoo,* Tahiti.
- *The Box,* Western Australia.
- *Third Dip,* Oahu, Hawaii.

Risks

It goes almost without saying that big-wave surfing can be extremely dangerous. For starters, the takeoff is critical. It's common for the board to catch a lot of air when dropping into large, steep, and hollow waves. This can easily result in the board becoming airborne . . . and its rider being sent to the bottom by several tons of speeding water. Large waves are also generally extremely fast; it's easy to get swallowed up and crushed by the falling lip. There are usually a lot of little ridges and bumps on the face of large waves, called *chop*, which can make merely standing a challenging endeavor. Finally, if you fall and end up in the impact zone, it's common to get held down for a little while. In cold water, a thirty-second hold-down can feel like five minutes! Depending on how you fall, you could easily head directly for the bottom, where contact with coral or rocks could result in serious injury, and even death.

To minimize these risks, big-wave surfers need to thoroughly prepare both physically and mentally. You must be extremely fit before you even think about paddling into large surf. And the progression to surfing the really big waves is best done through a very gradual comfort-zone expansion. Many experienced surfers are uncomfortable riding waves much larger than head high. As a result, they have no desire to ever take the risks that accompany big-wave surfing.

Limitations

Large waves, as noted, are usually very fast, and there's a point at which it isn't possible to paddle into them. There is also generally a limit as to the size of swell a break can handle. For example, a surf spot that is sweet at 10 feet could be *maxed out* or unsurfable at 15 feet.

Towing In

Tow-in surfing involves the use of a personal watercraft to catch waves that are too large to paddle into. The driver and rider take turns flinging each other into monstrous waves by means of a rope attached to the rear of the vehicle. The clearest advantages of towing rather than paddling are that you avoid getting air when dropping in and you can surf on a smaller, more maneuverable board.

Many purists in the sport reject the use of modern technology to catch large waves. Still, the largest waves have been ridden by towing in. Most big-wave surfers agree that there should be a progression to tow-in surfing. In order to safely tow in to gigantic waves, you need to first become proficient at pushing the paddle-surfing limits. Paddling into large waves is how you build your wave knowledge, skill, and confidence. As you become more comfortable, you can take off deeper. Paddle surfing a spot on a regular basis, when it's big, also gives you a chance to become accustomed to the impact zone and learn how to get yourself out of trouble. Tow in surfing is simply too dangerous if you're inexperienced, ignorant, and flung in a little too deep for your abilities.

Gear

Beyond having extreme skill, lots of nerve, and a penchant for severe risk taking, big-wave surfing also requires some specialized equipment. When gearing up, big-wave surfers need to take into account the wave size, wave shape, water temperature, and type of break. When surfers are equipped with a board too small for the conditions, they are said to be *undergunned*. This can possibly result in an inability to generate enough board speed or cause surfers to be bounced around excessively. If the board is too large for the waves, the surfer is *overgunned*. Riding waves with too large a board for the conditions might limit maneuverability or handling while surfing.

Gear Needed for Paddling into Big Waves

- A big-wave board usually between 9 and 10 feet.
- A big-wave leash usually around 12 feet.
- Wet suit, booties, gloves, and a hood, depending on the water and air temperature.

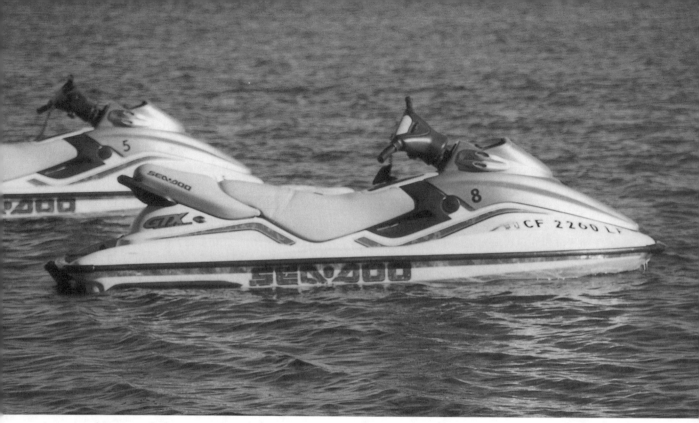

A personal watercraft for towing into big waves.

Gear Needed for Towing into Big Waves

- A tow-in board with straps usually around 7 feet.
- Wet suit, booties, gloves, and a hood, depending on the water and air temperature.
- A life vest.
- A towrope usually around 30 feet.
- A WaveRunner or other personal watercraft and trailer.
- A rescue sled.
- Gasoline.
- A lot of tools to work on the personal watercraft.

The Future

The number of athletes attracted to big-wave surfing has increased considerably in the last few years. This is a result of the sport experiencing a significant upsurge in attention, contests, and prize money.

As tow-in surfing becomes more popular, however, it also becomes more dangerous. On a huge day at some spots, you'll see multiple tow-in teams buzzing around. Things tend to get pretty unorganized. By all means observe the etiquette for towing in: Everyone hangs out on the shoulder and waits their turn. This will not only make the sport safer, but also save gas!

A Word to the Wise

Big-wave surfing is clearly not for everyone. There are numerous accomplished surfers who wouldn't even consider paddling out on a huge and unpredictable day. The bottom line is that surfers who are way out of their comfort zone will be a danger to themselves and others. If in doubt, just stay out!

Chapter 5

MANO a MANO Competition

The credit belongs to the man who is actually in the arena, whose face is marred by dust, sweat and blood. Who strives valiantly, who errors and comes short again and again. Who knows the great enthusiasms, the great devotion, and spends himself in a worthy cause and if he fails, at least fails while daring greatly. So that he'll never be with those cold and timid souls who know neither victory nor defeat. —*Theodore Roosevelt*

Surfing competitions may have originated as early as the 1500s somewhere in the South Pacific. Modern surfing competition, however, didn't really become popular until the 1960s in California. Since then, contests have been held at surf spots all around the globe, becoming an integral part of the surfing industry. As with any sport, surf-related product manufacturers use contests and athletes as vehicles to market their goods. Many surfing purists feel that competition clashes with the true spirit of the sport. They view surfing as an individual expression and soulful experience that is disserved by the commercialization of modern surf contests. Nevertheless, most agree that contests have contributed immensely to modern surfboard design and surfing technique.

Formats

Surfing contests have taken many different forms over the years. Some of the most common include longboard, shortboard, air, big wave, pro, amateur, collegiate, high school, and *grom* or *menehunes* (kids) contests. Contests can also differ in terms of the number of competitors per heat, the number of judges, and the way surfers are scored.

There are numerous contest tours at every level that hold events all over the world. Many contests schedule time frames or waiting periods in which the surfers are on standby to compete if conditions allow. Occasionally, a contest will be moved at the last minute to a venue that has better waves.

One of the most common formats is to have a few surfers go out and surf in a heat. For example, four surfers will go out for twenty minutes at a time, and only the two who score best will advance to the next round. There is generally a limit of ten waves that can be ridden by each athlete in the twenty-minute time period. Once a surfer's hands leave the board, the judges count that wave as one of the ten. Each competitor's best four waves will usually then be used to determine who will advance through the brackets to a final round of two surfers.

Contest day.

Pro Surfing

At the highest level of professional surfing competition, athletes are ranked internationally. The best-known organization for pro surfing, the Association of Surfing Professionals (ASP), ranks professional surfers worldwide.

Pro shortboard contests are held in places such as California, Hawaii, Brazil, Australia, South Africa, Japan, Europe, and Tahiti. Touring athletes travel extensively during the season and must constantly adapt to differing breaks and wave conditions. The best ASP shortboarders make competing a full-time job; their livelihood depends on prize money, photos, videos, and endorsements.

World Shortboard Champions

Year	Men	Women
1976	Peter Townsend	None awarded
1977	Shaun Tomson	Margo Oberg
1978	Wayne Bartholomew	Lynne Boyer
1979	Mark Richards	Lynne Boyer
1980	Mark Richards	Margo Oberg
1981	Mark Richards	Margo Oberg
1982	Mark Richards	Debbie Beacham
1983	Tom Carroll	Kim Mearig
1984	Tom Carroll	Freida Zamba
1985	Tom Curren	Freida Zamba
1986	Tom Curren	Freida Zamba
1987	Damien Hardman	Wendy Botha
1988	Barton Lynch	Freida Zamba
1989	Martin Potter	Wendy Botha
1990	Tom Curren	Pam Burridge
1991	Damien Hardman	Wendy Botha
1992	Kelly Slater	Wendy Botha
1993	Derek Ho	Pauline Menczer
1994	Kelly Slater	Lisa Anderson
1995	Kelly Slater	Lisa Anderson
1996	Kelly Slater	Lisa Anderson
1997	Kelly Slater	Lisa Anderson
1998	Kelly Slater	Layne Beachley
1999	Mark Occhilupo	Layne Beachley
2000	Sunny Garcia	Layne Beachley
2001	C. J. Hobgood	Layne Beachley
2002	Andy Irons	Layne Beachley

Judges

Surfing is a judged sport. As a result, there is an element of subjectivity in terms of what type of performance gets a good score. Each contest format has a certain set of criteria and maneuvers that the judges are looking for. Still, wave sizes and shapes dictate what maneuvers will be possible on any given day. There are usually enough judges at a contest to even out any biases and make events relatively fair. Judges take into consideration a variety of aspects of every competitor's surfing. A longboard judge might be looking for the length of a surfer's nose ride and the way the board is maneuvered. A shortboard judge might be impressed by how powerful or aggressive a maneuver off the lip is or by the length of a barrel ride. Regardless of the type of contest, most judges place a great deal of importance on technique and a surfer's style.

Technique

Surfing technique is, of course, constantly evolving. Every athlete can surf with a variety of different styles. Theoretically, however, there are relatively few body positions and weight transfers that constitute proper technique. Surfers' technique or the form they utilize in order to execute a turn or maneuver can carry a lot of weight with the judges. Expectations for technique in a contest will obviously rise with the level of competition.

As I've discussed in previous chapters, video analysis can be an incredible tool for competitive athletes to improve this aspect of their surfing. If

World Longboard Champions

Year	Men	Women
1986	Nat Young	None awarded
1987	Stuart Entwistle	None awarded
1988	Nat Young	None awarded
1989	Nat Young	None awarded
1990	Nat Young	None awarded
1991	Martin McMillan	None awarded
1992	Joey Hawkins	None awarded
1993	Rusty Keaulana	None awarded
1994	Rusty Keaulana	None awarded
1995	Rusty Keaulana	None awarded
1996	Bonga Perkins	None awarded
1997	Dino Miranda	None awarded
1998	Joel Tudor	None awarded
1999	Colin McPhillips	Daize Shayne
2000	Beau Young	Cori Schumacher
2001	Colin McPhillips	Cori Schumacher
2002	Colin McPhillips	Kim Hamrock

you want to improve specific elements of your performance you need to look at all aspects of it. Everything is interrelated. When you initiate a turn, you need to be aware of your body positions, where you're looking, and much more.

Along those same lines, every training session in or out of the water should have a purpose. If you're in the weight room or going for a run, you need to think about what you're trying to accomplish and develop a plan for how you're going to get there. Sometimes the objective when you're surfing might be to work on linking turns better or improving the consistency with which you successfully complete a difficult maneuver. One day you might concentrate on wave selection. The day before a contest, you might focus on just having fun. You'll find that there are times when it's useful to practice the art of not thinking about anything related to your technique at all. This can help you gain awareness of other aspects of your performance as well as serve to keep the sport enjoyable for you. The best way to transform your weaknesses into strengths is to consciously dedicate time, energy, and attention to improving them.

Regardless of how textbook your form is, judges might penalize you if you're unable to link turns smoothly or project a sense of energy in your ride. This, ladies and gentlemen, is where the style element enters the equation.

Style

Style is an elusive concept that's difficult for anyone, including judges, to quantify. All surfers have a unique style that evolves throughout their careers. The best surfers in the world have a style that can adapt to the conditions, format, competitors, or what the judges are looking for. Within every type of surfing, you'll find surfers with dif-

fering styles. Some are more fluid, seeming to make long, drawn-out lines in the wave. Others surf with more energy, as if they're one with the wave in each maneuver. The most successful contest surfers are usually those who can marry the two to create a unique and exciting performance.

Judges tend to reward surfing that looks effortless but pushes the envelope of what's possible. This means that a surfer who can fluidly link multiple radical maneuvers in a single ride will often score well. Judges like to watch a surfer who seems to be in complete control of the wave but is also taking huge risks. As a result, contest surfers need to have an idea of which maneuvers they'll perform, keeping in mind that safe, within-yourself surfing usually won't win. To come out on top, an athlete must be willing to attempt difficult maneuvers in critical parts of the wave that may have a low rate of success. On the flip side, however, life is so sweet if you pull it off!

Wave Selection

One of the most important factors in surf contests is wave selection. Competitors can give themselves the best chance for scoring well by choosing waves that will help showcase their surfing style. A combination of years of contest experience and knowledge of a specific break can help surfers select the biggest, best-shaped, or somehow best-suited waves in a set for the way they surf. At a big-wave contest, for example, it's important to be able to read the swell direction to maximize your chances of selecting a large wave that won't close out.

We improve our wave-selection skills every time we surf. Each session results in a little more ocean knowledge and wave experience. Still, in a contest it's important to be able to assess an incoming swell very quickly. And depending on how much time is left in the heat and how well you think you've scored up to that point, you can decide whether or not to get into position for a particular wave. Sometimes you can afford to patiently wait for the near-perfect wave; other times you'll be forced to take a marginal wave and make it work.

Priority

The term *priority* is used in contests to describe one surfer having precedence or the choice of wave over another surfer during a heat. This can be granted before the heat to a surfer who has won a coin toss or scored highest in previous rounds. Priority can also be determined during the heat by which athlete has paddled past a certain point or buoy first.

Having the choice of wave can be a tremendous advantage, especially on a day when waves are inconsistent or small. Surfers with priority can choose the best waves in a set and leave their competitors struggling to score well on marginal waves. This can force the athlete without priority to attempt more radical maneuvers in order to catch up.

Interference

In contests, dropping in on another surfer is called *interference*. The judges view this as a serious infraction and will penalize the surfer who has dropped in. The athlete whose ride has been interfered with will very likely not be pleased either!

Fatigue

Fatigue can play a decisive role in the latter rounds of a contest. By the time surfers have advanced to the semifinals or finals of an event, they may have already surfed in four or five heats

that day. This can result in athletes becoming tired both physically and mentally. To combat this, it's important to be well conditioned, stay hydrated, and stay out of the sun between rounds. We'll talk about conditioning in great depth in the chapters that follow.

Heat Dynamics

As with any type of competition, surf contests have a unique set of dynamics. Most contests pit surfer against surfer in heats of four. The dynamic of the four surfers in each heat can vary from amiable to hostile depending on the type of competition, what's at stake, conditions, and past experiences among the athletes. Each surfer wants to score as many good waves in a heat as possible. So things can get ugly if surfers don't follow some basic etiquette. It's common for visiting, less experienced competitors to feel intimidated by aggressive local veterans. In amateur, one-day events, surfers may not interact much at all. Some surfers may not have met one another before the contest and may not see each other again for the rest of the season. But in tours where surfers compete against each other throughout the year, it's much more common for friendships and rivalries to develop.

Coaching

Coaching is a relatively new concept in the competitive surfing world. One reason I started coaching surfers is that I saw so many great athletes with so little direction. There were surfers with loads of talent but little knowledge of what they could be doing to take their skill to the next level.

As a surfing coach, I believe that you cannot separate the needs of the athlete from the needs of the person. Any stresses that you experience

Recent ASP Shortboard World Champion Vitals

Source: www.aspworldtour.com, May 2002

Female

Layne Beachley
World Champion: 1998–2002
Date of Birth: May 24, 1972
Place of Birth: Sydney, Australia
Years Rated: 13
Stance: Regular
Height: 5' 5"
Weight: 125 pounds
Career Earnings: $382,335

Lisa Anderson
World Champion: 1994–1997
Date of Birth: March 8, 1969
Place of Birth: Florida
Years Rated: 13
Stance: Regular
Height: 5' 6"
Weight: 128 pounds
Career Earnings: $303,860

Pauline Menczer
World Champion: 1993
Date of Birth: May 21, 1970
Place of Birth: Sydney, Australia
Years Rated: 15
Stance: Regular
Height: 5' 3"
Weight: 121 pounds
Career Earnings: $356,305

Male

C. J. Hobgood
World Champion: 2001
Date of Birth: July 6, 1979
Place of Birth: Florida
Years Rated: 6
Stance: Goofy
Height: 5' 7½"
Weight: 148 pounds
Career Earnings: $245,433

Mark Occhilupo
World Champion: 1999
Date of Birth: June 16, 1966
Place of Birth: Sydney, Australia
Years Rated: 19
Stance: Goofy
Height: 5' 9"
Weight: 194 pounds
Career Earnings: $682,263

Kelly Slater
World Champion: 1992, 1994–1998
Date of Birth: February 11, 1972
Place of Birth: Florida
Years Rated: 11
Stance: Regular
Height: 5' 9"
Weight: 160 pounds
Career Earnings: $827,055

Sunny Garcia
World Champion: 2000
Date of Birth: January 14, 1970
Place of Birth: Honolulu, Hawaii
Years Rated: 16
Stance: Regular
Height: 5' 10"
Weight: 200 pounds
Career Earnings: $861,580

away from the sport—work, school, family—will impact your athletic performance. I am convinced that the most effective way to prepare is to follow a periodized training program that incorporates individual goals, strengths, weaknesses, and time constraints.

There are no quick fixes. Change of any kind takes time, whether physical, technical, or psychological. Sporadic physical, technical, or mental preparation provides little benefit. It is commitment, hard work, and patience that enable athletes to make the necessary adaptations to enhance their athletic performance. It has been my experience that surfers must follow a periodized and individualized training program consistently for at least six months before change becomes fully ingrained.

I work with surfers in training and competitive environments to improve the physical, technical, and mental aspects of their performance. I learn a great deal about individual athletes and how to enhance their performance through talking and working out with them, analyzing video and training logs, as well as attending their surf sessions and contests. I emphasize variety, fun, goal setting, and education. Athletes who understand why they do what they do have a tendency to commit more fully to their training and subsequently obtain better results.

It is necessary to take a "big-picture" view of athletic development. Physiological, technical, strength, and psychological improvements are made more efficiently when periods of training volume, intensity, and recovery are cycled. The different elements of a total training program must have cohesion and a common purpose in order to maximize time and energy and achieve optimal performance.

This book has been written with this coaching philosophy and approach in mind. My goal is to equip you with the knowledge you need in order to take your surfing to the next level. We become empowered by intelligently educating ourselves about all aspects of surfing performance. In other words, I want you to be able to take the information presented in this book and couple it with your own experience to eventually coach yourself.

Perspective

Most surf contests are a lot of fun. The majority of athletes don't take themselves too seriously and tend to keep things in perspective. If a bigger event is held close to a populated area, the organizer can expect a decent spectator turnout. This helps increase the amount of energy at a contest and contributes to the already positive vibe. After all, win or lose, the surfers are doing something they love—and perhaps taking home some money or products at the end of the day, too!

Chapter 6

FUEL Nutrition

Never believe you have insufficient time for the attention to detail that is essential to excellence. You have exactly the same twenty-four hours every day as Carl Lewis, Magic Johnson, and Evander Holyfield. —*Dr. Michael Colgan, author of* Optimum Sports Nutrition

Now that we've discussed what we can do in the water to enhance performance, it's time to look at other factors that can have a significant impact on the way we surf. As most of us know by the way our stomachs grumble shortly after a long, consistent session, we expend a lot of energy when we surf. Our bodies need energy to enable us to do everything from paddling out during an epic storm swell to staying warm on a frigid day.

There are a variety of different opinions and definitions of what *proper nutrition* means. Simply put, food is fuel, and the more active you are, the more important your nutrition. In other words, what you ingest directly affects your physical performance. As the quote that opens this chapter points out, maximizing human potential and athletic performance requires taking every possible factor into consideration.

The three major categories of fuel are carbohydrates (bread, pasta, fruit . . .), proteins (meat, eggs, beans . . .) and fat (cheese, oil, butter . . .). The amounts and ratios your body requires of each depend on your individual needs.

For the most part, surfers need a higher percentage in their diets of carbohydrates than of fat

and protein. During a session, we burn a lot of our glycogen stores, which carbohydrates can replace. Fat is a great energy source and an important part of everyone's diet, but the majority of us eat a lot more than our bodies need. Protein is essential for helping build or rebuild muscle tissue, but is also generally overeaten. If you were to break things down, average avid surfers would want roughly 45 to 60 percent of the calories they consume to come from carbohydrates, 20 to 35 percent to be derived from protein, and 10 to 25 percent to come from fat. Where each person falls within that range depends on numerous factors related to individual energy needs.

Energy Needs

We differ in our physical activity, body compositions, and physiology. The amount, frequency, and type of exercise we get also play a large role in our energy demands. For example, marathon runners generally require a higher percentage of carbohydrates and a lower percentage of protein than sprinters. A person's weight and percentage of lean muscle mass are also determining factors. If two people weigh the same, the one who pos-

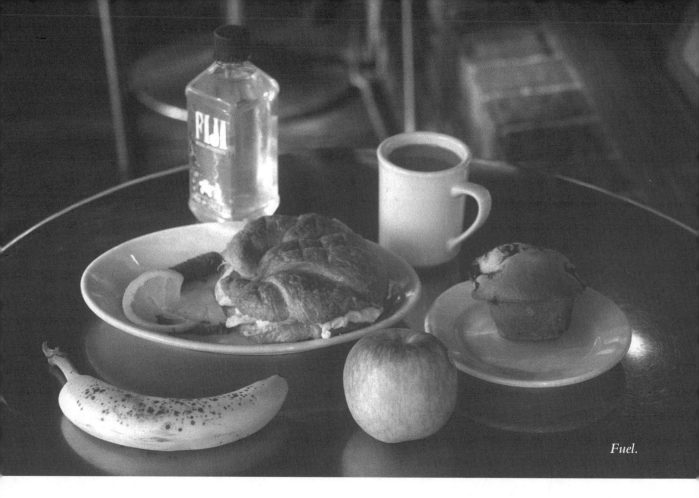

Fuel.

sesses a higher percentage of lean muscle mass will burn more calories just sitting on the couch. Lastly, genetics and metabolism dictate nutritional needs. Some people need to eat all day in order to maintain their weight while others can seemingly gain weight by simply thinking about food.

Many competitive athletes keep track of what they eat and drink in a training log. This can allow them to identify patterns and better understand their energy needs and the relationship between what they ingest and their performance.

Weight

While we're on the subject of nutrition, we might as well discuss weight. Our body mass, or what we weigh, is directly related to our body composition. *Body composition* refers to the per-

centages of our mass that are made up of things like bone, organs, fat, muscle, and other soft tissue. You can change your mass by gaining or losing fat and lean muscle through changes in diet and exercise.

Surfing requires a unique compromise between flexibility and power. Overall, your ideal total weight as a surfer will be determined not by your percent of body fat and lean muscle mass but also by your height, weight, age, gender, surfing style, and the types of waves you surf. In general, you don't want to weigh so much that you're slow and inflexible, or so little that you get bounced around by the slightest chop.

Muscle is denser than fat and therefore weighs more. For example, you could lose a significant amount of body fat, gain some muscle mass, and still weigh the same. Thus, weight alone isn't a great indicator of fitness. It's more important to determine an athlete's body fat and lean muscle mass percentages.

Body Fat and Lean Muscle Mass

Because surfing requires power and a high strength-to-weight ratio, it's best to have a relatively low body fat percentage. Having low body fat will minimize the amount of dead weight resisting you during a long paddle, a quick pop-up, or a big air. Still, having too low a body fat percentage can decrease your energy level, ability to recover from an injury, and immune response.

Body fat percentage is the percent of total body mass that consists of fat. Sports medicine specialist Jack Wilmore, of the University of Arizona, recently reviewed more than one hundred studies on body composition. His analysis shows that the body fat of elite athletes ranges from 4 to 16 percent for males and 8 to 25 percent for females, depending on the sport. My experience has been that the majority of serious competitive surfers seem to perform best at between 5 and 9 percent for men, 14 and 18 percent for women. Again, please note that your optimal body fat percentage is extremely individual and will be influenced by factors such as the types of waves you surf, surfing style, age, activity level, genetics, and percentage of lean muscle mass.

Lean muscle mass percentage is the percent of total weight that is made up of muscle. As surfers, we require a high strength-to-weight ratio. In other words, we are most concerned with relative strength or strength in relation to our body weight. In order to be powerful, we need to be quick as well as have a high strength-to-weight ratio. If we are carrying too much fat or muscle, we tend to move slower, lose flexibili-

ty, and consequently compromise the amount of power we can generate.

Athletes tend to vary greatly in their percentage of lean muscle mass in large part due to the demands of their sport. A sprinter or football running back will generally carry a higher percentage of lean muscle mass than a tennis player or marathon runner. I've observed that most surfers perform best when their lean muscle mass percentage falls somewhere in the middle of the spectrum.

Determining Body Composition

There are numerous ways to determine your body composition. The most common, easily accessible, and inexpensive techniques are skin fold measurements and electric current analyzers. Skin fold measurements involve the use of calipers to pinch the skin in certain areas of the body. Electric current analyzers use electrodes placed on the hands and feet to measure the amount of resistance encountered between two sites. The results for both methods are then calculated taking into consideration a person's age, gender, height, weight, and activity level.

If you're interested in seeking out either of the above methods for determining body composition, you might have to call around a little, depending on where you live. Most health clubs and physical therapy offices have calipers for skin fold measurements. Be sure to ask for the most qualified personnel at the facility, however, because human error is common with this technique. Some health clubs, physical therapy offices, and university human performance labs have electric current analyzers.

More expensive and accurate methods for analyzing body composition are hydrostatic weighing and the use of a machine called a Bod Pod. These are usually found in university laboratories, research facilities, or private physical performance institutes that offer lab testing for athletes. Hydrostatic weighing involves submerging the subject in a tank of water. Because fat tends to float and muscle sink, the weighing device can determine body composition more precisely. A Bod Pod looks like a large hollow egg in which the subject is enclosed. This machine can accurately determine body composition by measuring volume displacement and by combining it with other data entered into a computer.

Hydration

Most people are constantly a little dehydrated. Most of us have heard the recommendation that the average person should drink twelve eight-ounce glasses of water each and every day. The more active you are, the more water you need to drink throughout the day to keep an ideal amount of fluid in your body. As activity, air temperature, and the dryness of the air increase, so too does the demand for water.

Hydration is important to surfers because dehydration means a loss of blood volume. Lower blood volume means a loss of power. The blood supplies muscles with oxygen and nutrients. If there is less blood in your body, it takes longer for muscles to get the oxygen they need during exercise. This delay could mean a decrease in strength, endurance, and power, which can in turn have a negative impact on performance.

Having less water in muscle tissue can also decrease performance. According to a study done by M. Sawka and published in the *Journal of the American Medical Association* in 1984, a muscle that's dehydrated by only 3 percent can cause a 10 percent loss of contractile strength and an 8 percent loss of speed. In other words, we can avoid significant decreases in power, since

strength and speed are the two elements of power, by staying well hydrated.

Surfing hard on a warm day when the air is dry can quickly lead to a significant loss of water in the system. Fluid is lost through the skin in the form of sweat as well as during respiration.

Sweating is the body's way of cooling itself. The amount you sweat when you're active depends on how strenuous the activity is, air temperature, air humidity, body composition, physiology, and whether or not you're accustomed to exercise. Remember, just because you're in the water doesn't mean that you're not sweating and becoming dehydrated.

We also lose vital minerals and electrolytes such as salt and potassium through our sweat. As a result, many athletes use an energy replacement drink, rather than just water, to hydrate before, during, and after strenuous exercise. There are numerous products on the market. Avoid sports drinks that contain high levels of simple sugars like glucose or sucrose because they inhibit absorption of water by your body. The gas in carbonated drinks like soda also slows down absorption. Fructose/glucose polymer drinks work best because they contain fewer carbohydrates and small amounts of certain minerals that have been shown to enhance fluid absorption.

A simple way to help replenish what is lost through perspiration during the day is to drink diluted fruit juice. At first, the taste may not appeal to you, but after a while most people grow to prefer drinking juice diluted by at least 50 percent. In general, juice is bottled in concentrations too high for your body to maximally absorb its water as well as the various vitamins and minerals.

We also lose water from our body when we breathe. With every exhalation, moisture is lost to the atmosphere. When the air is dry, this water is not replaced by the next inhalation. Even if all you're doing is just sitting still and breathing, you could become significantly dehydrated within a few hours.

I'm not proposing bringing a water bottle into the water with you; I'm merely stressing the importance of hydrating before and after your sessions as well as throughout the day. A good rule of thumb is to start hydrating a few hours before a hard workout, surf session, or contest. Drink an eight-ounce glass of water every fifteen minutes starting four hours before the event and stopping twenty minutes before strenuous exercise to avoid bladder issues. Be sure to sip rather than gulp in order to avoid swallowing a lot of

air, which can disturb stomach function and slow absorption.

Simply put, staying well hydrated will help maximize performance as well as aid in basic physiological functions. Most of us wouldn't think of driving around with too little coolant in their car's radiator, but we often never think twice about keeping our own systems hydrated.

Diuretics

Diuretics are substances that draw water from your system. The most commonly ingested diuretics are alcohol and caffeine. Drinking diuretics can lead to dehydration, and, as I discussed earlier, dehydration can result in a loss of power. One of the most common dehydration

Average Water Temperatures in the United States
Source: The National Oceanographic Center

	Jan	Feb	Mar	Apr	May	Jun	Jul	Aug	Sep	Oct	Nov	Dec
San Juan, P.R.	77	78	78	79	80	81	81	83	83	82	81	80
Oahu, Hawaii	76	76	76	76	78	79	80	80	81	81	79	77
St. Petersburg, Fla.	62	64	68	74	80	84	86	86	84	78	70	64
San Clemente, Calif.	57	57	58	58	60	63	65	68	66	64	61	58
Santa Cruz, Calif.	53	54	54	54	55	56	58	59	60	59	56	54
Ocean City, Md.	37	34	42	49	55	62	68	71	70	62	53	44
Newport, Oreg.	49	50	50	50	52	55	55	55	56	54	53	52
Anchorage, Alaska	31	31	32	34	44	54	58	57	53	44	34	32

scenarios is drinking a few beers the night before a surf session and then downing some coffee the next morning to fire up your system. When you drink little or no water in combination with this routine, you're sure to be very dehydrated. This will affect your ability to quickly paddle outside for a set wave or carve a powerful arc off the shoulder.

Supplements

The use of dietary supplements has become increasingly popular among athletes. In my opinion, most of us won't notice a significant benefit to our performance by using a lot of the supplements out there that we wouldn't see from eating well and staying well hydrated. It seems that for every supplement produced, there are several opinions as to how it should be used. Keep in mind that many factors play a role in a supplement's effectiveness.

What follows are brief descriptions of a few of the most common supplements being used. My intent is to merely give you some examples of the type of supplements that are available and in no way promote their use. If you're contemplating using any kind of supplement, you should research its effectiveness and side effects. It's also advisable to consult your physician or other qualified health professional to maximize your safety.

- *Caffeine.* Caffeine is found in coffee, tea, cocoa, caffeinated sodas, and chocolate and has had a reputation for years as an effective performance enhancement supplement. Studies have shown that taken in the right amounts, caffeine increases adrenaline release, stimulates the central nervous system, and helps us utilize body fat as fuel, which aids in the conservation of glycogen. As I've noted, however, because caffeine is a diuretic, using it as a

supplement should be done carefully. One study conducted on cyclists by Dr. Lars McNaughton in Australia showed that ten milligrams of caffeine per kilogram of body weight taken three hours before exercise allowed the athletes to ride both longer and harder. On the other hand, research has also shown that if you already habitually use it, no amount of extra caffeine will benefit you. And still other studies deny that it will aid performance for anyone.

- *Creatine.* Creatine phosphate, commonly known as just creatine, is a high-energy phosphate compound that is used by your body to rapidly resynthesize adenosine triphosphate (ATP), an immediate source of energy for muscle contraction. Creatine has become an increasingly popular supplement among athletes. There seems to be some evidence that it can help decrease the amount of recovery time needed after exercise. It has also been shown to cause cells to retain more fluid, giving the appearance of greater muscle mass. Often this fluid is lost within a week or two of discontinued use. Creatine is now available in many different forms, and there are conflicting studies and opinions as to whether it will enhance performance.

- *Ginseng.* Ginseng is an herb derived from three different plants and has been a supplement popular among endurance athletes. There are numerous types of ginseng, and many have been proven to (among other things) increase an athlete's use of body fat as an energy source. There are also experts in the field of sports nutrition who are of the opinion that ginseng will not benefit athletes whatsoever.

- *Glucosamine.* This is a building block used by the body to manufacture specialized molecules called glycosaminoglycans, found in cartilage. It's been used as a supplement by a lot of injured athletes in a variety of sports. There is some evidence that it can help with the healing of ligament, tendon, cartilage, and muscle tears.

- *L-Carnitine.* L-Carnitine is a substance that is made by the body and used to transport fat. It's a supplement that has been used for years. Some research studies have concluded that it can enhance anaerobic and aerobic performance.

- *Multi-vitamin and mineral supplements.* These supplements are very common and appear to be most beneficial to people who have difficulty eating a well-balanced diet. Overdosing on fat-soluble vitamins such as A, D, E, and K can be toxic and thus hazardous to your health. Water-soluble vitamins such as vitamin C can be taken in very large amounts and will likely only result in perhaps diarrhea or the production of fluorescent and expensive urine!

Health

Whether you're a competitive surfer or just starting out, it's good to know how what you consume can affect your physical performance. I'm not proposing that you take the fun out of eating and overanalyze your nutritional needs constantly. There's no need to become obsessive—just aware, knowledgeable, and responsible. The more in tune you are with what your body needs, the better you'll be able to perform at your highest level consistently. Still, the most important reason to treat your system well nutritionally is to ensure that you'll be healthy enough to surf for the rest of your life. After all, what good is retirement if you can't do what you love?

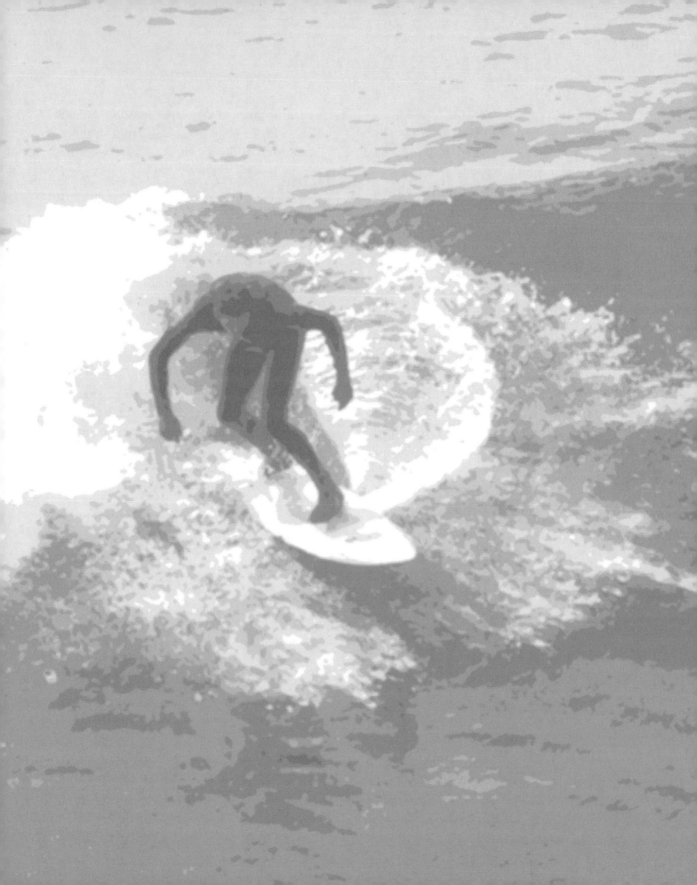

Chapter 7

GUMBY Flexibility

Excessive muscular tension tends to decrease sensory awareness of the world and raise blood pressure. —*Larson and Michelman, 1973 study*

Optimal movement requires flexibility. In order to get into and maintain certain body positions, it's imperative that you're not only strong and stable but also flexible. For example, if you've ever gone to a yoga class, you know that it takes a lot more energy for a novice to get into and hold even the most basic of poses than it does for someone who has been practicing yoga for years. Well, the same holds true in surfing. An inflexible surfer is more prone to injury and has a more difficult time popping up fluidly, crouching, kneeling, or rotating than a flexible surfer. The more active you are, the more important it is that you stay flexible.

Injury Prevention

Some of the most common surfing injuries are sprains and strains in the foot, ankle, knee, lower back, shoulders, and neck. All of these types of musculoskeletal injuries can be minimized or prevented by increasing flexibility. Being strong with stable joints does you very little good in terms of injury prevention if you're inflexible. Stretching can help reduce stress on joints and allow them to handle greater forces without suffering significant trauma. In all sports, flexible athletes are less likely to get injured, and strong athletes who don't stretch are usually the first to

get injured. This is because as people gain muscle mass, they generally need to stretch more frequently in order to maintain their flexibility.

Besides injury prevention, maintaining your overall flexibility is an important element of surfing performance. Specifically, we as surfers need to stay limber in order to effectively pop up, get into low positions, and rotate.

Popping Up

The pop-up needs to be a fluid and often explosive motion. Even the strongest of people would have a difficult time going from their bellies to their feet in one motion on dry land if they were very inflexible. Getting your feet underneath you while still keeping your hips low takes above-average flexibility of the lower body.

Getting Low

There are many occasions in surfing when you need to lower your center of gravity by dropping your hips. If you're unable to squat without your heels coming up, then you're automatically in a less stable position, because all your weight is now on the balls of your feet. Or if the only way you can get under the lip is to bend over at the waist, as opposed to dropping your hips, then you've compromised your stability and strength.

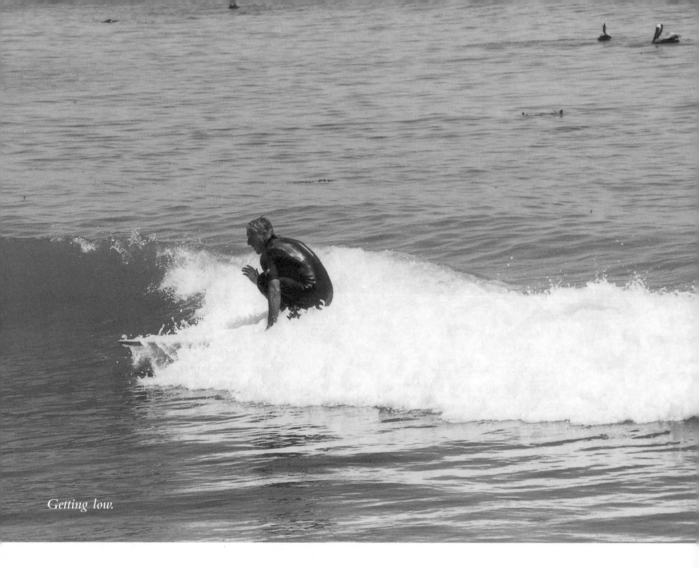

Getting low.

Your center of gravity is now significantly farther forward. If you've ever flipped through a surfing magazine, you've probably noticed that a lot of the smaller barrel photos require a surfer to be low and stretched out on the board. Some of these positions could be yoga poses in and of themselves! Moving smoothly and effortlessly on land is a prerequisite to fluid movement on a speeding surfboard.

Rotation

In surfing, a lot of power is generated through rotation. Stiff surfers who don't have full range of motion in their upper bodies and hips are quite simply less powerful than they could be. Have you ever held the bottom of a spring and twisted the top? If so, you probably noticed that there was a lot of energy produced when you let go of one end of the spring. Well, the human spine is similar. All of the muscles, ligaments, and tendons that attach vertebrae to vertebrae and the spine to the pelvis need to stay flexible in order to maintain full range of motion and to maximize rotational power.

Basic Kinesiology

The muscles that are most important for surfers to stretch are labeled in the following illustrations.

Surfing muscles, front view

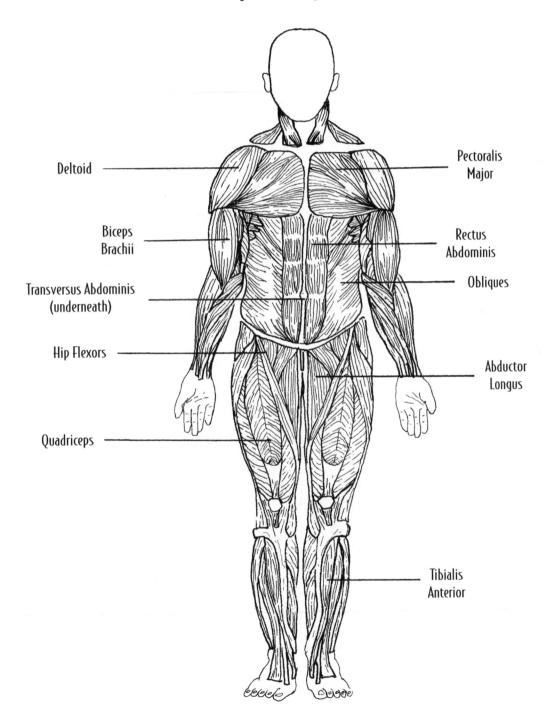

Deltoid

Pectoralis
Major

Biceps
Brachii

Rectus
Abdominis

Transversus Abdominis
(underneath)

Obliques

Hip Flexors

Abductor
Longus

Quadriceps

Tibialis
Anterior

Surfing muscles, back view

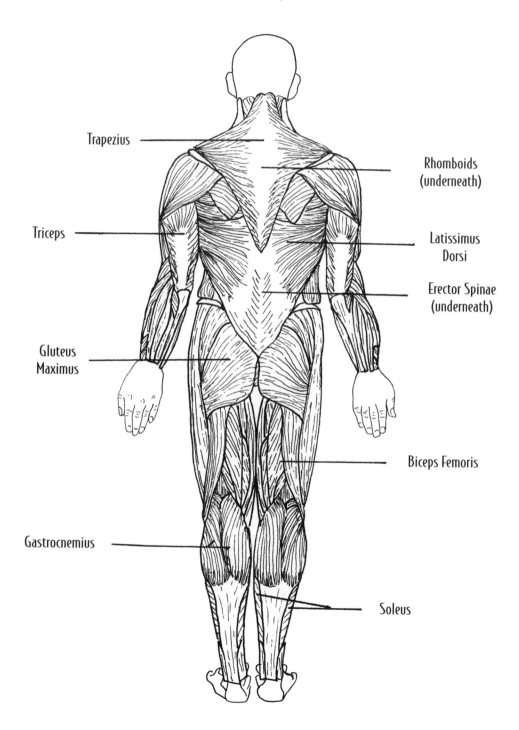

Trapezius

Rhomboids
(underneath)

Triceps

Latissimus
Dorsi

Erector Spinae
(underneath)

Gluteus
Maximus

Biceps Femoris

Gastrocnemius

Soleus

Main Paddling Muscles

- *Biceps brachii (bis).* Located on the front of the upper arm.
- *Deltoids (delts).* Shoulder muscles.
- *Latissimus dorsi (lats).* Attach at the back of the upper arm and fan down the back.
- *Rhomboids.* Located between the shoulder blades.
- *Trapezius (traps).* Attach on the back of the skull and fan down the shoulders.
- *Triceps brachii (tris).* Located on the back of the upper arm.

Main Trunk Stabilizers Used in Surfing

- *Erector spinae (back extensors).* Run along length of the spine.
- *Internal and external obliques.* Run at angles across the midsection.
- *Rectus abdominis (abs).* Run vertically along the front middle of the midsection (aka six-pack).
- *Transversus abdominis (T.V.A.).* The body's natural weight belt, it goes around the mid-section.

Main Pop-Up Muscle

- *Pectoralis major (pecs).* Run along the chest.

Lower-Body Muscles Used in Surfing

- *Adductor longus (adductors).* Run along the inner thigh.
- *Gastrocnemius and soleus (calves).* Run behind the lower leg.
- *Gluteus maximus (gluts).* The large and powerful buttock muscles.
- *Biceps femoris (hamstrings).* Run behind the upper leg.
- *Hip flexors.* The various muscles around the hips that allow you to bring your knees up.

- *Quadriceps (quads).* The various muscles that run on the front of the upper leg.
- *Tibialis anterior (tibs).* Run along the front of the shin.

When and How to Stretch

Even relatively sedentary people should make a habit of stretching at least five to ten minutes per day. Active individuals and athletes should spend five to ten minutes stretching lightly before exercise, and ten to fifteen minutes of deeper stretches after exercise. All stretching will be safer and more effective if it follows at least five minutes of light to moderate aerobic exercise. This will increase blood flow to the musculature and result in greater elasticity. People who are genetically less flexible will need to spend more time and energy stretching to become flexible. And as we get older, most of us will need to commit more time to stretching in order to maintain our flexibility.

There are two main ways to stretch: passively and actively.

Passive stretches, the most common, are those stretches that are deepened slowly, gradually, and in a controlled manner. A passive stretch should be held for between ten and thirty seconds, depending on how tight the muscle is and the desired goal of stretching. It's also helpful to take full, slow, and deep breaths while stretching passively. This will make the experience more relaxing for you and allow you to deepen the stretch slightly with each exhale. Passive stretches can be done before and after exercise.

Active stretches, which are much more advanced, involve taking muscles and supporting soft tissue to full ranges of motion during specific movements. Stretching actively requires above-average flexibility, joint stability, and body awareness. Examples of active stretches would be a walking-forward or lateral lunge, or throwing a two- to three-pound medicine ball against a trampoline. The advantage of this type of stretching is that you can increase the amount of blood flow to soft tissue while you stretch. This makes active stretching most beneficial when performed before a workout, because it can enhance your preparation for exercise. On the other hand, it's more difficult to control a stretch when it's done actively, which in turn will increase the risk of injury while stretching. As a result, I make sure the athletes I work with stretch actively only under my supervision, and once I'm thoroughly convinced that their bodies are prepared to meet the demands of the movement.

Stretching should not be painful, be too strenuous, or involve jerky or bouncing movements. The last thing you want to do is injure a muscle that you'll need in the water! It's also important not to overstretch. Your goal is to increase or maintain flexibility in order to improve range of motion, regain symmetry, and enhance performance. Stretching beyond a muscle's capability can eventually lead to compromised stability and function.

Yoga

Yoga classes and videos can be a very effective way to increase your flexibility. Be cautious, however, with poses that go beyond the stretching capabilities of the muscle. Such positions can actually stress joint capsules and supporting tendons and ligaments. This may in turn lead to joint instability and/or inflammation. In order to utilize yoga safely and effectively, you'll want to do some research and seek out instructional videos, books, or classes that match your goals, needs, wants, and abilities. As with anything, think critically about what you're trying to accomplish. If you're practicing yoga with the goal of improving your surfing, then you probably won't need to go to extremes.

Massage

Many types of massage can help keep muscles flexible by lengthening and increasing blood flow to tissue. Getting massages on a regular basis can also release toxins and lactic acid from the muscles and aid in recovery. A lot of high-level athletes in a multitude of sports use massage as a way to help keep both their muscles and their minds relaxed. I recommend finding a licensed massage therapist who works with athletes and is within your price range. Massage services at spas, for example, tend to be costly and not geared toward the needs of athletes. Pre-event massages, within forty-eight hours of a contest, should be relatively light and invigorating. Deeper massages can be very beneficial as well, but these can cause temporary muscle soreness and as a result are best performed two to three days before an exceptionally strenuous workout or event.

Stretching Exercises

What follows are some passive stretches that can be easily done at home, in the gym, or at the beach. How deep a stretch is taken and the amount of time it is held will depend on your degree of flexibility and your needs as a surfer.

Passive Stretching Exercises

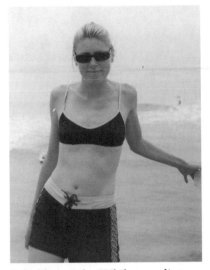

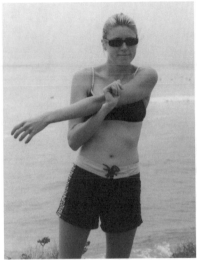

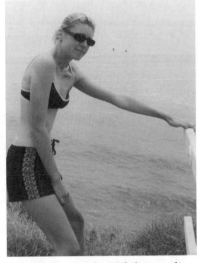

Deltoid stretch. *While standing, hold on to something and lean forward while keeping your arm bent.*

Lat stretch. *Pull your arm straight in front of your body and pull your elbow with the opposite arm.*

Rhomboid stretch. *While standing and holding on to a fixed object, pull away from the object and turn your torso.*

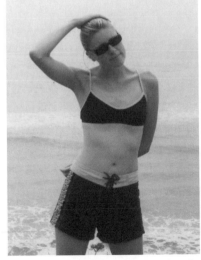

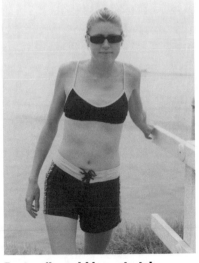

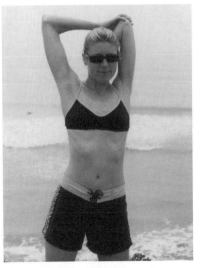

Trapezius stretch. *Pull your head forward and to the side with one hand while your opposite hand is behind your back.*

Pectoralis and bicep stretch. *While standing, hold on to something and lean forward while keeping your arm straight.*

Tricep stretch. *Bring your arm above your head and pull on your elbow with the opposite arm.*

Passive Stretching Exercises (continued)

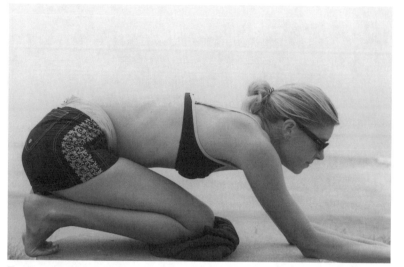

Back extensors. *While kneeling, flex your spine forward and push your weight back onto your feet.*

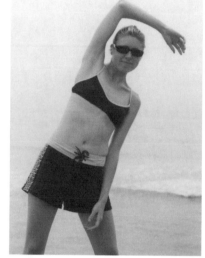

Oblique stretch. *While standing with a wide stance, flex your spine laterally.*

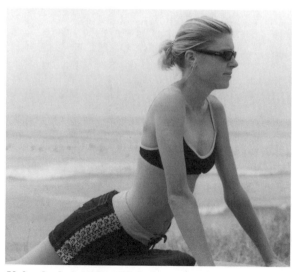

Abdominal stretch. *While lying facedown, arch your upper body up by pushing with your arms.*

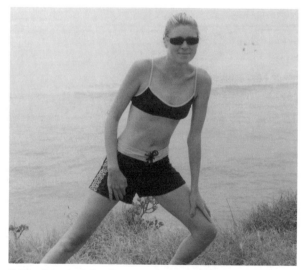

Adductor stretch. *From a lateral lunge position, put more weight on one leg, keeping the opposite leg straight.*

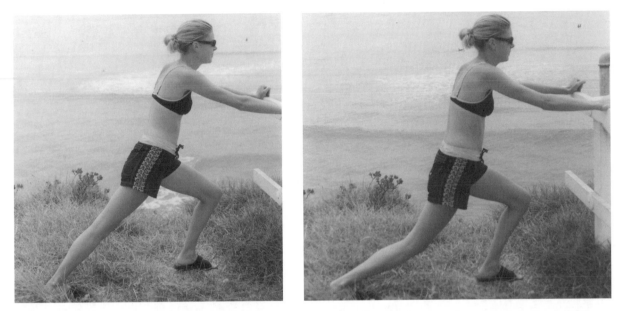

Calf stretch. *Lean your upper body forward, keeping your feet flat on the ground, and stretch first with your knee straight (left) and then flexed (right).*

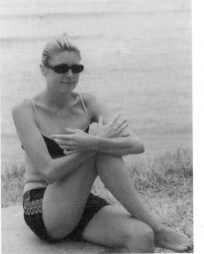

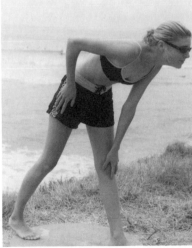

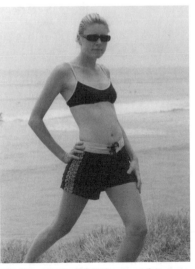

Gluteus stretch. *While sitting, pull one knee toward the opposite shoulder.*

Hamstring stretch. *Put your hand at hip level, keeping one leg straight and the other leg back, then bend forward at the waist.*

Hip flexor stretch. *From a lunge position, push your hips forward.*

Passive Stretching Exercises (continued)

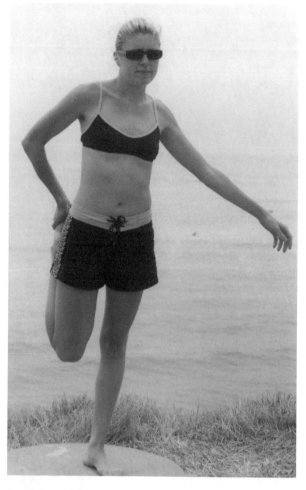

Tibialis anterior stretch. *While standing, roll your toes underneath your foot and lean forward.*

Quadriceps stretch. *Pull your heel to your butt while standing.*

As You Age

Flexibility generally decreases as we get older. Therefore, we need to dedicate more time to stretching as we age merely to maintain our muscle elasticity. This is due to a variety of factors but is accelerated when people are sedentary and neglect their bodies. As a result, staying flexible will not only help you surf better but will help keep you feeling young!

Chapter 8

CARDIO Aerobic and Anaerobic Fitness

Pain is weakness leaving the body. —*The Marines*

The term *cardiovascular fitness* refers to how accustomed your heart and lungs are to exercise. This is important because working muscles require oxygen in order to contract effectively. And muscles that work better help surfers increase safety, enjoyment, and performance. Unconditioned surfers are hazards to both themselves and others. There are moments when it's imperative to keep paddling in order to get back outside or avoid another surfer. Cardiovascular fitness can also help you recover more quickly between efforts and catch more waves during your session. From a performance standpoint, however, this element of fitness is essential: It's the foundation for strength, power, agility, stability, and skill development. If you think of your overall fitness as a pyramid, cardiovascular exercise would be the broad base. Without such a foundation, you'll be unable to build your conditioning pyramid to its maximal potential.

There are two main types of cardiovascular exercise: aerobic and anaerobic. *Aerobic* exercise is physical activity performed at an intensity at which your heart and lungs are able to deliver adequate oxygen to working muscles. The primary energy source of prolonged aerobic efforts is fat. *Anaerobic* exercise is physical activity in which your heart and lungs are unable to meet the oxygen demands of the musculature involved, creating an oxygen debt. Because fat can only be "burned" in the presence of oxygen, the primary energy source of anaerobic activity is glycogen. Glycogen is the storage carbohydrate that's unique to mammals. The largest reserves of this energy source can be found in our muscles, making it a readily available fuel.

Aerobic Capacity

Aerobic capacity refers to a person's ability to sustain a medium-intensity aerobic effort for extended periods of time. For example, a surfer who has a high aerobic capacity will have an easier time paddling to an outside break, holding position when the current's strong, and moving around in the lineup when the peak is shifting. Developing a high capacity for aerobic activity means that your lungs can get a good deal of oxygen into the bloodstream quickly and your heart is effective at pumping this oxygenated blood to working muscles. Simply put, increasing aerobic capacity is the first step in developing overall fitness. A high aerobic capacity will improve endurance and is required in order to achieve better anaerobic endurance.

How to Improve

Aerobic capacity can be improved through prolonged, medium-intensity aerobic activity.

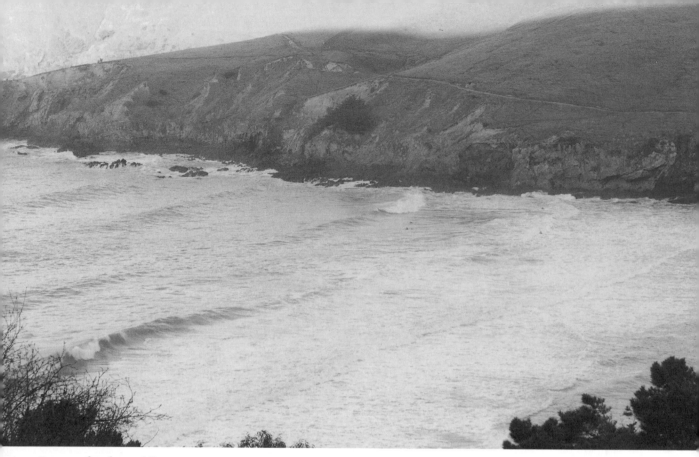

Prepare for the paddle out.

Endurance sports such as swimming, running, and cycling are very effective in developing aerobic capacity. Ocean swimming is one of the best aerobic activities, because being comfortable and proficient at dealing with currents and open-water waves could help you one day when you're surfing.

Of course, ocean swimming is also appreciably more dangerous than doing laps in a pool. You not only need to deal with waves and currents but also have to take into consideration factors such as water temperature, wildlife, and boats. When swimming in a pool, you can hop out if you get tired or cold. That's obviously not always an option during an open-ocean swim. I recommend wearing a wet suit that's designed for open-water swims and choosing days when there's little or no current in areas that are pro-

tected from significant wave action. This will make it easier to stay relatively close to shore where there are fewer boats, and safer in the event that you need to exit the water quickly. Aerobic workouts should last at least thirty minutes and be performed above 55 percent of your maximum heart rate and below your anaerobic threshold.

You've probably heard that your maximum heart rate can be found by subtracting your age from 220. This doesn't hold true for everyone, but it can give you a ballpark number with which to estimate where your heart rate should be for aerobic and anaerobic workouts. You can also find your maximum heart rate by wearing a heart rate monitor during a hill sprint or stair workout. For example, after a twenty- to thirty-minute warm-up, find a steep hill or long flight of stairs to run up. If you run as fast as you can up that hill or flight of stairs for ten seconds and then walk down, your maximum heart rate should register two to three seconds after you finish the fourth or fifth sprint. Such a heart rate test is very strenuous, however, and should only be attempted by well-conditioned athletes.

The *anaerobic threshold* (A.T.) is the point at which the muscles go into oxygen debt and lactic acid, the by-product of metabolizing glycogen, is produced more quickly than it can be cleared from working muscles. As a result, lactic acid concentration increases and creates an acidic environment that makes it difficult for the muscle to contract. This is also the point at which working muscles and lung musculature will start to feel as if they're "burning" and fatigue quickly. Exercise that's performed above the anaerobic threshold results in improving *lactate tolerance* (L.T.), or the ability for working muscles to contract in a more acidic environment. This type of

training will also train the body to adapt to the stress by becoming more efficient at clearing lactic acid from working muscles.

The anaerobic threshold for most surfers is reached between 80 and 90 percent of their maximum heart rate. For example, if your max is 200 beats per minute (bpm), then your A.T. will probably be somewhere between 160 and 180. You'll probably feel this same "burn" after you've been running at a comfortable, relaxed pace on flat ground for a while and then attempt to maintain the same speed up a hill. This is your anaerobic threshold, and if you were wearing a heart rate monitor you'd find that your heart rate would be between 80 and 90 percent of your maximum. Thus, aerobic activity meant to improve aerobic capacity should be performed below this point, at a heart rate between 55 and 80 percent of your maximum heart rate.

What follows are heart rate ranges or zones that correlate to aerobic and anaerobic workouts.

Heart Rate Zones for Optimal Fitness

Heart Rate Zone	Workouts
55–70% of your maximum heart rate	Long aerobic workouts designed to burn mostly fat
71–83% of your maximum heart rate	Aerobic interval training to improve A.T.
84–92% of your maximum heart rate	Anaerobic interval training to improve L.T.
93–97% of your maximum heart rate	Anaerobic work to improve maximal oxygen uptake
98–100% of your maximum heart rate	Sprint workouts to improve maximal efforts

Aerobic Interval Training

Interval training is a type of energy system workout that involves periods of intensity followed by rest. It allows more work to be performed at higher exercise intensities with the same or less fatigue as continuous training. Interval training can be done while hiking, in-line skating, ocean or river kayaking, outrigger canoeing, mountain biking, paddle boarding, road cycling, running, or swimming.

Aerobic interval training will help increase your anaerobic threshold. Having a high anaerobic threshold will allow you to go relatively hard for extended periods of time before you go into oxygen debt. As a result, you'll be able to recover more quickly between efforts and have more energetic surf sessions. When the waves are good, your conditioning should not be a limiting factor in how many waves you catch.

Aerobic intervals are relatively painless and are most effective when done between five and ten beats per minute below the anaerobic threshold. As we discussed before, for most active people the A.T. is between 80 and 90 percent of your max heart rate. It's better to err on the side of a little too easy than a little too hard: Once you've reached A.T., you're no longer training to increase the threshold but are training muscle lactate tolerance, or your muscles' ability to contract in a more acidic environment. In other words, if you've reached the point of lung and muscle burn, you've gone too hard.

Aerobic interval sessions should last from thirty to ninety minutes total, with individual intervals lasting from one to ten minutes and rests of three to six minutes in between.

Anaerobic Endurance

Anaerobic endurance is your ability to sustain a high-intensity anaerobic effort for relatively short periods of time. For example, the 100-meter and 400-meter track events in running utilize the anaerobic energy system, whereas a marathon primarily makes use of the aerobic energy system. In other words, folks with good anaerobic endurance are able to use glycogen as an energy source efficiently, and their muscles are trained to contract in a more acidic environment. When we surf, anaerobic endurance is needed for those one to five minutes of hard paddling to get out of the impact zone. We also use this energy system for accelerating the board in order to catch waves, get out of another surfer's path, or get outside for a big set.

Anaerobic Interval Training

Anaerobic interval training will help increase muscle lactate tolerance. As a result, working muscles will be able to contract in a more acidic environment and won't fatigue as quickly. This is important for those very intense, short bursts of energy required to get to a safe spot, catch a wave, or connect multiple, powerful maneuvers on a single wave. The last thing you want to do is run out of gas during a contest or when the waves are powerful and have good shape.

Anaerobic intervals are shorter and more painful than aerobic intervals. These intervals are done above the A.T. and are accompanied by a great deal of lung and muscle burn. An anaerobic interval session might also last from thirty to ninety minutes. Each interval might be thirty seconds to two minutes in length with one to five minutes of rest in between.

Sample Thirty-Minute Aerobic Interval Session (Easy)

Activity	Intensity	Heart rate
10-minute warm-up	Low	55–65% of max
1½-minute aerobic interval	Medium	5–10 bpm below A.T.
2-minute recovery	Low	55–65% of max
2-minute aerobic interval	Medium	5–10 bpm below A.T.
3-minute recovery	Low	55–65% of max
1½-minute aerobic interval	Medium	5–10 bpm below A.T.
10-minute cool-down	Low	55–65% of max

Sample Sixty-Minute Aerobic Interval Session (Difficult)

Activity	Intensity	Heart rate
15-minute warm-up	Low	55–65% of max
4-minute aerobic interval	Medium	5–10 bpm below A.T.
4-minute recovery	Low	55–65% of max
5-minute aerobic interval	Medium	5–10 bpm below A.T.
4-minute recovery	Low	55–65% of max
5-minute aerobic interval	Medium	5–10 bpm below A.T.
4-minute recovery	Low	55–65% of max
4-minute aerobic interval	Medium	5–10 bpm below A.T.
15-minute cool-down	Low	55–65% of max

Sample Thirty-Minute Anaerobic Interval Session (Easy)

Activity	Intensity	Heart rate
10-minute warm-up	Low	55–65% of max
45-second anaerobic interval	High	Above A.T.
3-minute recovery	Low	55–65% of max
1½-minute anaerobic interval	High	Above A.T.
4-minute recovery	Low	55–65% of max
45-second anaerobic interval	High	Above A.T.
10-minute cool-down	Low	55–65% of max

Sample Sixty-Minute Anaerobic Interval Session (Difficult)

Activity	Intensity	Heart rate
15-minute warm-up	Low	55–65% of max
1-minute anaerobic interval	High	Above A.T.
3-minute recovery	Low	55–65% of max
1½-minute anaerobic interval	High	Above A.T.
4-minute recovery	Low	55–65% of max
1-minute anaerobic interval	High	Above A.T.
3-minute recovery	Low	55–65% of max
1-minute anaerobic interval	High	Above A.T.
15-minute cool-down	Low	55–65% of max

Another type of anaerobic interval training is a sprint workout. These consist of very short, all-out intervals. Such training is designed to overload you or to improve your ability to give maximal efforts and recover between them. Sprints utilize what's called the adenosine triphosphate–creatine phosphate (ATP–CP) energy system. This is an energy source that can be used very rapidly by working muscles but is also in very limited supply. As a result, each sprint should last around ten seconds and should be followed by two to five minutes of rest, depending on your goal. Since a sprint workout is effectively over once you're unable to get your heart rate well above your anaerobic threshold, five to ten sprints should suffice. Sprint workouts are very strenuous, specialized workouts that should only be attempted after you're very well conditioned.

The above workouts are very structured and will be most effective when performed with the use of a heart rate monitor. Still, if you're pretty well in tune with your body and have a good sense of how hard your heart and lungs are working, you can also go by feel.

As with any physical activity, it's important to ease yourself into interval training. Start with very short intervals and a lot of rest, and then gradually progress. Because it's easy to burn out on this type of training program both physically and mentally, make sure you've thought through when it fits within your program. I'll discuss how to incorporate workouts like intervals into a training program in chapter 14. I want to point out, however, that regardless of your goals, structured interval training should happen no more than once a week in order to avoid fatigue and overtraining.

Here's an example of how aerobic and anaerobic workouts might fit into a weekly training program in the off season.

Weekly Workouts for the Off-Season

Monday	Off
Tuesday	60 min. surf / 40 min. strength training / 10 min. trunk stability / 10 min. stretch
Wednesday	90 min. surf / 30 min. interval training / 15 min. stretch
Thursday	40 min. aerobic workout / 10 min. trunk stabilization / 10 min. stretch
Friday	30 min. balance and agility workout / 15 min. stretch
Saturday	60 min. surf / 45 min. strength training / 15 min. stretch
Sunday	90 min. surf / 30 min. aerobic workout / 15 min. trunk stability / 15 min. stretch

Cross-Training

Cross-training is a term used to describe the workout activities that athletes perform other than their own sport. And it's a must for both the recreational and the competitive surfer. There are three reasons why.

First, surfing alone will not allow you to reach your fitness potential. Although surfing can be a great workout, its energy demands are inconsistent and unpredictable. You can't control the frequency or size of the sets. In other words, to a great extent you have no power over the demands that will be placed on your energy systems or musculature. One day, for instance, you might get a lot of rest between efforts because the waves are marginal. Another day your heart rate might be up during the entire session due to constantly fighting the current just to hold your

Cardio Cross-Training Options

Activity	Surfing Elements Incorporated
Beach volleyball	Aerobic, agility, anaerobic, endurance, power, strength
Hiking	Aerobic, anaerobic, endurance, strength
In-line skating	Aerobic, agility, anaerobic, balance, endurance, strength
Ocean kayaking	Aerobic, endurance, ocean knowledge, strength, trunk strength
Outrigger canoeing	Aerobic, anaerobic, endurance, ocean knowledge, strength, trunk strength
Mountain biking	Aerobic, anaerobic, balance, endurance, power, strength
Paddleboarding	Aerobic, anaerobic, balance, endurance, power, strength
River kayaking	Aerobic, anaerobic, endurance, strength, trunk strength
Road cycling	Aerobic, anaerobic, balance, endurance, power, strength
Running	Aerobic, anaerobic, endurance, strength
Swimming in the ocean	Aerobic, anaerobic, endurance, ocean knowledge, strength, trunk strength
Swimming in a pool	Aerobic, anaerobic, endurance, strength, trunk strength

position in the lineup. As a result, relying on surfing alone to get fit isn't the most effective way to maximally improve a lot of the physical elements you need to surf, such as flexibility, strength, power, endurance, aerobic capacity, and anaerobic endurance.

Second, as with any skill sport, bad habits are created when you're fatigued. Using surfing as your only means of getting into shape can lead to poor habits in the water, which may take a great deal of time to correct.

Third, prolonging surf sessions so that they're more of a workout can lead to fatigue that can impair judgment and increase risk of injury.

Keep It Fun

Cardiovascular fitness is the base of the health and wellness pyramid. Once aerobic exercise becomes a part of your weekly routine, it shouldn't take a whole lot to maintain your endurance. The high-end work, on the other hand, takes a great deal of motivation and commitment to sustain. That said, vary your cardiovascular training activities so that you don't start to dread every workout. Whatever your goals may be, getting your heart rate up should be fun. Otherwise you'll be less likely to stick with it in the future!

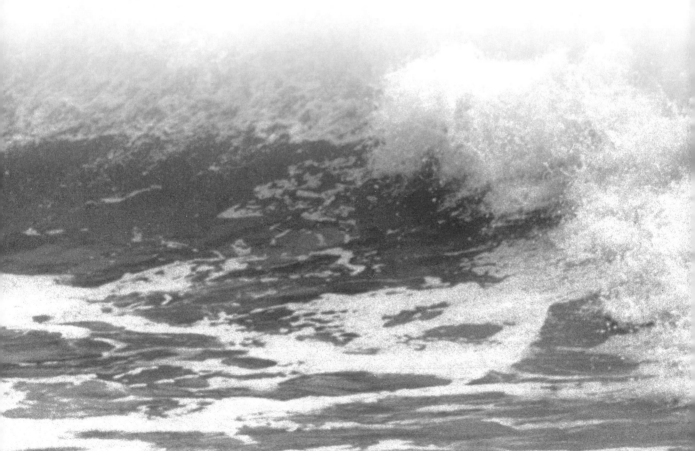

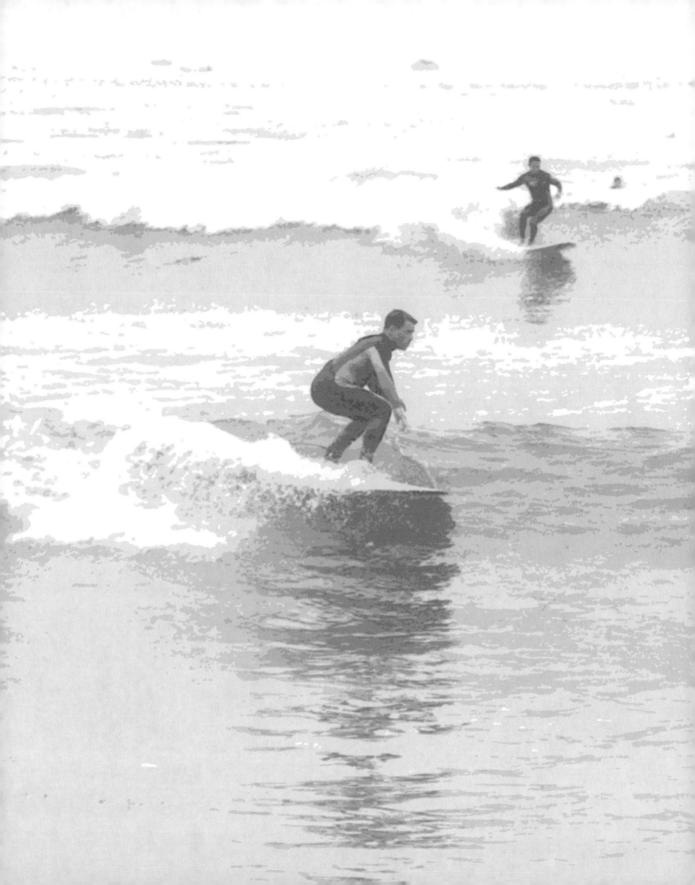

Chapter 9

FAST TWITCH Agility and Quickness

The faster you do things, the less accurate you become. —*Fitt's Law*

Agility and quickness are essential elements of surfing performance. Many of the movements you make with your feet, ankles, knees, and hips when you surf happen with a great deal of precision and speed. As with any skill sport, as a surfer you need to contract a number of small and large muscles surrounding each joint that's involved in a maneuver, in varying amounts. Your body recruits these muscles in response to factors such as speed changes, gravitational forces, and water resistance. You have to make constant adjustments in this muscle recruitment throughout a series of linked maneuvers. When done well, surfing performance looks fluid, powerful, and athletic.

You need to be agile or precise in your weight distribution so as not to overcompensate in reaction to forces that are exerted upon you. Consider the analogy of driving on a dirt road. If you take a corner too fast and the back end of your car begins to slide, you want to turn the steering wheel in the direction of the skid. Yet you only want to turn it as much as you need to get the vehicle back to center. If you overreact and turn the wheel too far, you'll send the back end sliding in the opposite direction. Similarly, when we're releasing or applying pressure to one rail of our board, we make small adjustments to muscles all the way from our feet to our neck. In

order to roll our ankles, knees, hips, and torso into a new turn, we need a multitude of muscles to coordinate their contractions very quickly, in just the right amount, to execute the desired movement.

The two components of agility are coordination and speed. As we know, the faster we attempt to perform a movement, the less precise we become. If we train correctly, however, we can improve our quickness and agility. As surfers we can also create adaptations in our nervous system and musculature by performing drills on land that will increase our accuracy at higher speeds. This will directly translate to greater agility in the water.

Fast- and Slow-Twitch Muscle Fibers

As humans, we possess two types of muscle fiber: slow twitch and fast twitch. *Fast-twitch fibers* are activated during all-out exercise requiring rapid and/or powerful, anaerobic movements. In contrast, *slow-twitch fibers* are recruited to sustain continuous, aerobic activities. In surfing, as in most sports, we use both muscle fiber types. For example, we primarily utilize slow-twitch fibers during a long paddle and fast-twitch fibers if we paddle hard to catch a wave.

Why is this important? Well, research has shown that through training we can alter the composition of our musculature to meet the demands of our particular sport. In other words, sprinters can train to increase the percentage of fast-twitch muscle fibers in their legs, and marathon runners can increase the percentage of slow-twitch in theirs. Now, of course, there are genetic limitations to how much we can alter muscle composition, but nevertheless it can be changed. This means that if we want to improve our surfing performance by becoming quicker and more agile, we can train our muscles in such a way as to eventually increase the amount of fast-twitch musculature we have at our disposal.

Drills

Any drill to improve quickness and agility should be functional. In other words, you should be able to relate it to surfing movements and performance in some way. This is relatively easy because our sport is so dynamic that we need to train virtually every muscle in our bodies to help us become more agile. Instead of giving you a list of agility drills that I use with the athletes I work with, I urge you to do some brainstorming of your own. It's been my experience that athletes are more apt to enjoy agility and quickness training if they play a role in creating the workouts. So what follows are lists of variables to consider and of equipment ideas.

There are numerous variables you should take into consideration when developing agility drills designed to improve your surfing. I don't expect every drill you come up with to be entirely sport specific. The idea is that, as I've mentioned throughout this book, you think critically about what and why you're doing something in an effort to get the best possible results. The objective is to train your body to be prepared beyond the demands placed on you by

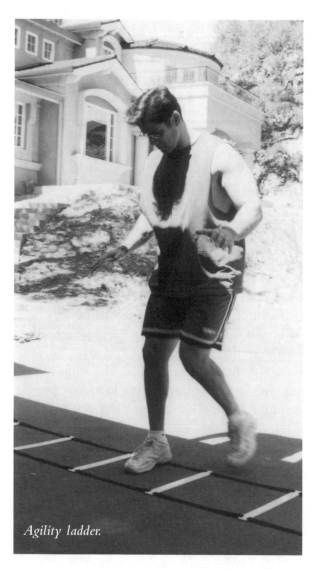

Agility ladder.

your surfing, while still keeping things relatively safe. You want to perform drills as quickly and accurately as possible while also promoting proper body positions and biomechanics.

Agility Drill Equipment Ideas

- *Jump rope.* Great for warming up. It can be used in an agility drill: Try to jump precisely over a line or into squares drawn on the ground with chalk or created with masking tape.

- *Agility ladder.* This is a ladder made usually of plastic and nylon and placed flat on the ground. It can be used for a multitude of different one- and two-legged jumping, hopping, or quick-stepping drills.
- *Hurdles.* These are usually made of plastic and vary in height from 6 to 18 inches. They can be used for various one- and two-legged jumping or hopping drills alone or in conjunction with an agility ladder.
- *Cones.* These vary in height and can be used for a multitude of different one- and two-legged jumping, hopping, quick-stepping, or running drills.
- *Tape.* Tape is great for making different-length lines or shapes on the ground that you have to jump or step over or into with one or two legs.
- *Boxes.* You need boxes of varying heights that can support your weight. These are usually referred to as plyometric boxes and can be used for a multitude of different one- and two-legged jumping, hopping, or quick-stepping drills alone or with other boxes.
- *Full foam rolls.* These are dense Styrofoam rolls that you can roll forward or backward like a log. They promote fast feet and are great for challenging the small, fast-twitch muscle fibers in the foot and ankle.
- *Hackysacks.* Picture small beanbags that you can juggle with anything but your hands; great for promoting eye–foot coordination and fast reactions. They're most fun with two or three other people.
- *Reaction balls.* These small, odd-shaped rubber balls bounce unpredictably when thrown on hard surfaces and are great for improving reaction times and overall quickness and agility.
- *Medicine ball.* This is a heavy ball that you can use to increase the difficulty of almost any

agility and quickness drill. Try holding the ball in front of you to promote a quiet upper body, for instance, or playing catch with someone else while your feet are performing a particular drill.

Agility Drill Variables That Can Be Manipulated

- *The length of the drill and duration of the workout.* Quickness and agility won't improve if you're fatigued; each drill should be relatively short—ten to thirty seconds—and the whole workout should take between twenty and sixty minutes.
- *The three planes of movement used in surfing.* These are the frontal plane (lateral movements); the sagittal plane (flexion and extension); and the horizontal plane (rotation up to 360 degrees).
- *Varying the drills in your workouts.* As with anything, your body will adapt to specific movements; you need to continually challenge your musculature and nervous system by mixing things up.
- *The range of motion required of the drill.* Since surfing is dynamic, the range of motion required during a drill can be dynamic.
- *The limbs, muscles, and joints involved.* Sport specificity in this area means a higher likelihood of the drill improving your surfing.
- *The muscle contraction required.* For example, your legs contract both concentrically and eccentrically when you surf—concentrically when you extend your legs, and eccentrically when you flex your knees.
- *The coordination of body parts during a drill.* You'll want to keep your upper body stable and quiet during certain drills that involve you being quick with your feet, ankles, knees, and hips.

- *The intensity of the movement.* For example, a drill requiring you to hop on one leg is more intense than the same drill done while hopping on both legs at the same time.
- *The perceptual skills incorporated into your drills.* Since surfing requires you to look ahead and constantly assess situations, some of your drills should also incorporate and challenge these skills.
- *The energy system demands incorporated into your agility workouts.* Certain exercises should place a similar demand on your heart and lungs as does surfing.

Cross-Training

Although structured agility and quickness workouts are extremely effective, you can also train these surfing elements through certain cross-training activities. This will help keep you from getting burned out on the drills you've created and can just be plain fun!

Overall Athleticism

Improving your agility and quickness will undoubtedly result in enhanced surfing performance—but at the same time will also promote overall athleticism. In general, the more athletic you are, the better you'll be able to perfect new maneuvers and adapt to things such as changes in wave shape, wave size, wave speed, and equipment. As I've noted before, the best way to take your surfing to the next level is to challenge yourself beyond the demands of what surfing confronts you with.

Agility Cross-Training Options

Activity	Surfing Elements Incorporated
Alpine skiing	Aerobic, agility, anaerobic, balance, power, strength
Basketball	Aerobic, agility, anaerobic, endurance, power, strength
Beach volleyball	Aerobic, agility, anaerobic, endurance, power, strength
Racquetball	Aerobic, agility, anaerobic, endurance, power
Skateboarding	Aerobic, agility, anaerobic, balance, power, strength
Snowboarding	Aerobic, agility, anaerobic, balance, power, strength
Soccer	Aerobic, agility, anaerobic, endurance, power
Tennis	Aerobic, agility, anaerobic, endurance, power
Wakeboarding	Agility, anaerobic, balance, power, strength
Waterskiing	Agility, anaerobic, balance, power, strength

Chapter 10

STABILITY Balance

Balance is a highly integrated and dynamic process that involves multiple neurological pathways.... For example, a relatively simple activity such as sprinting ... requires losing and regaining your balance on one leg in less than 1/10 of a second. —*Michael A. Clark, MS, PT, PES, CSCS,* *author of* Integrated Training for the New Millennium

The sport of surfing may be the ultimate practice of dynamic balance. (*Dynamic*: constantly changing; *balance*: a relative state to the position or movement of your body over the board.) The wave is always moving and changing shape. A surfer needs to react quickly to changes in board speed and angle. Surfers of all abilities need to have stellar balance in order to accelerate the learning curve. Complex surfing maneuvers start with the ability to make constant, subtle adjustments in body position. This requires a well-trained nervous system that can quickly recruit the musculature needed to stabilize the spine, pelvis, and involved joints. Often the limiting factor in progression in the sport is a balance deficiency that is due to lack of flexibility and/or stability. In essence, if you want to improve, you need to train your balance dynamically.

Balance and Trunk Stability

Dynamic balance is dependent on trunk stability—the ability to coordinate the muscles in your abdomen and back with specific movements. Since your center of gravity is below and behind your navel, the better you can stabilize

your pelvis and spine, the better you'll be able to control the majority of your weight.

The point at which your spine meets your pelvis is essentially the largest joint in the body. In surfing, it's often necessary to maintain a certain postural position and/or keep your hips and shoulders level in order to best execute a turn or maneuver. This creates a strong foundation for movement and makes it easier for joints such as ankles, knees, hips, and shoulders to be stabilized.

Trunk musculature such as the transverse abdominis, internal obliques, external obliques, rectus abdominis, erector spinae, and latissimus dorsi (see the illustrations on pages 91 and 92) all work together to stabilize the spine and pelvis. Thus, an effective way to reach your dynamic balance potential is to train these muscles with specific exercises that involve stabilizing your torso.

Balance and Joint Stability

Dynamic balance is also very dependent upon joint stability. *Joint stability* refers in part to the integrity, flexibility, and strength of the muscles, tendons, and ligaments that provide movement

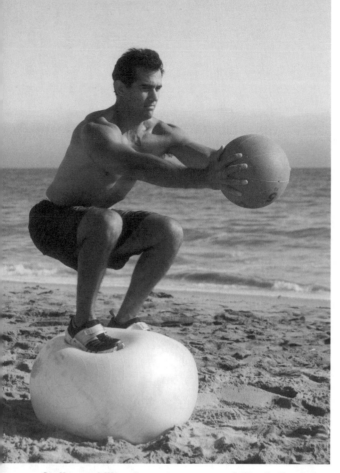

Stellar stability. *Squatting on a stability ball while holding a medicine ball.*

for a joint. At the same time, stability also requires the ability of the nervous system to recruit the right amounts from each muscle, large and small, in order to control movement of the joint.

If you can stabilize your trunk and joints quickly and effectively, you'll more than likely have what we would call good balance. In our sport, it's important to develop full body strength, flexibility, symmetry, and stability. As I've said earlier, trunk stability provides the foundation for movement. Stellar trunk strength and stability makes it easier to control the positions of your joints because it helps keep your center of gravity relatively quiet. If, however, you're unable to keep

your ankles from rolling in and your knees from knocking, you'll probably have a tough time even executing a proper bottom turn.

Therefore, it's important to realize the effect an unstable joint can have on your balance and consequently your surfing. For example, a strained or sprained ligament in an ankle or knee will result in a less flexible, weaker, and less stable joint. This can in turn lead to a loss of symmetry between the left and right sides of the body, which will affect your ability to quickly recenter after a cut back or keep your feet under you when landing a big air!

Athletic Stance

As previously mentioned, balance starts with a strong athletic stance. This can also be described as your ready position—the position that allows you to stay over the board at all times. From this stance, you are ready for just about anything the wave has to offer. This position should be relaxed and comfortable, allowing for the variety of movements your body will make. An athletic stance varies somewhat from individual to individual. Still, almost everyone's body position should include feet shoulder width apart; more weight on the balls of the feet; a bend in the ankles and knees; a slight drop in the hips; chest up, with a natural and slightly forward spine position; hands out in front with elbows slightly bent; relaxed shoulders; head level to the ground to allow the eyes to look ahead.

You can find your athletic stance by jumping up in the air with your eyes closed a few times. Each time you land, take note of the position your body naturally relaxes into. Try to find that position more quickly with every jump. After a few jumps, open your eyes and analyze your stance. You should feel light on your feet, with

Athletic Stance

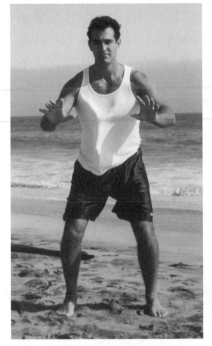

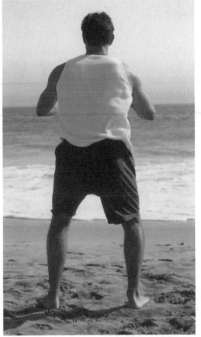

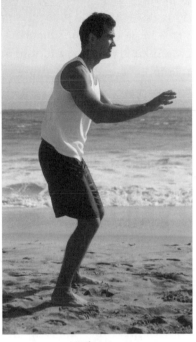

Front view   *Rear view*   *Side view*

your center of gravity low, balanced, and ready to move in any direction.

Knee Tracking

The term *knee tracking* refers to the position of the patella or kneecap in relation to the foot during movement. This is important because if the knee is tracking too far to one side or the other, it can place undue strain on the ankle, knee, and hips during movement. This can ultimately result in an increased risk for injury and/or a loss of stability, strength, and power. The most biomechanically advantageous knee tracking position for most people is directly over the second toe—the one next to your big toe. This position provides most of us with the best platform to maximize strength and power.

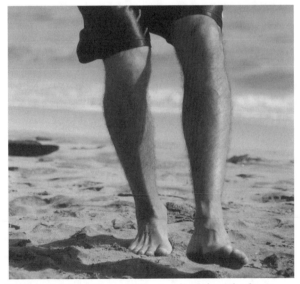

Knee tracking. *The patella is aligned with the second toe during flexion.*

Deviations too far left or right of the optimal knee tracking position rely too heavily on tendons, ligaments, and muscles rather than bony structures as a base of support.

Ankle stability and foot structure play a large role in knee tracking. If your tendency is to pronate—to roll in your foot and ankle—then your knee will more than likely follow. Conversely, if your tendency is to supinate, or roll your foot and ankle outward, then your knee will tend to track outward. Your goal is to maintain as neutral or evenly weighted a foot position as possible. Some athletic shoes are made to help correct for one tendency or the other. A neutral foot position, however, needs to become habitual or automatic—when you're surfing, that's one of the last things you'll be thinking about!

Instability of the ankles, knees, or hips and lack of flexibility in any muscle of the lower body can also affect the way the knee tracks. For example, imbalances in strength or flexibility in the muscles of the hip joint can alter the position of the femur, which will directly affect the position of the knee.

Stability Training Exercises

The beauty of stability training is that you can do many of these exercises several times a week without ever really feeling fatigued. Many athletes in dynamic balance sports will train their balance in fifteen- to thirty-minute workouts three or four times per week. Often, athletes will train for stability and agility in the same workout on days that they aren't strength training. And since these workouts don't need to be very strenuous, they can be done on a recovery day or the day before a contest.

Again, you'll find it easier to stabilize if you maintain an athletic stance and use your trunk musculature to stay centered. It's also helpful to focus your eyes on a point at least a few feet in front of you and at eye level to keep your head up. The following exercises should be done in a safe area and only after a good warm-up and a light stretch.

Dynamic Balance Strength Training

Once you've mastered a dynamic balance exercise, one way to increase its difficulty is to introduce a strength component. For example, when kneeling on a stability ball becomes easy, you can grab a couple of dumbbells and do arm curls while you're on the ball. As a result, a single exercise can integrate and improve dynamic balance, trunk stabilization, *and* strength. Surfers at every level can also benefit from squatting on an unstable surface. For instance, doing squats to a ninety-degree bend in your knees while standing

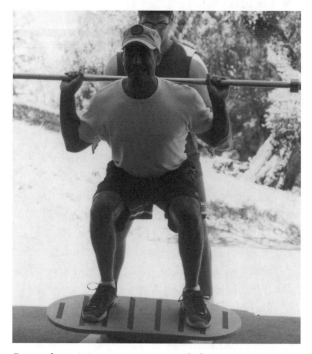

Strength training on a rotating balance trainer.

Basic Balance Exercises

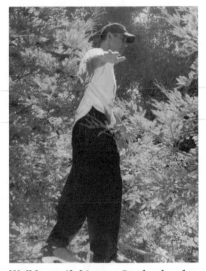

Walking a tightrope. *Look ahead; stabilize your pelvis with your trunk musculature; keep your hands in front of your body.*

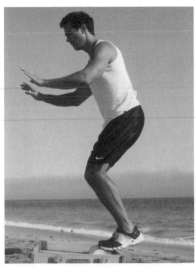

Standing with your feet on the edge of a step, eyes closed. *On the balls of your feet, focus on maintaining perfect posture; keep your ankles relaxed to make small and quick adjustments.*

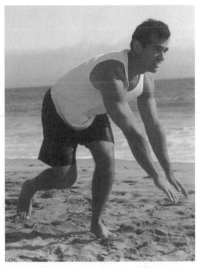

Bending at the waist at different angles while standing on one foot. *Maintain a neutral spine; keep a slight bend in your knee; keep your knee tracking over your second toe.*

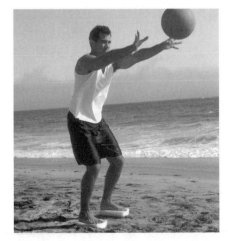

Standing on half a foam roll and tossing a medicine ball. *Maintain an athletic stance, relaxed ankles, and soft knees; toss and catch the ball, using your trunk muscles to stabilize your pelvis and spine.*

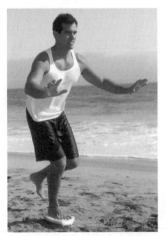

Standing on one leg on half a foam roll. *Keep a slight bend in your knees and relaxed ankles; minimize your upper-body movement.*

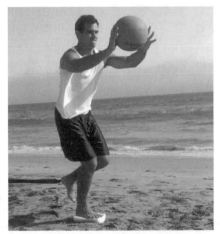

Standing on one leg on half a foam roll and tossing a medicine ball. *Keep a slight bend in your knees and relaxed ankles; toss and catch the ball with minimal upper-body movement; stabilize your pelvis and spine.*

Basic Balance Exercises (continued)

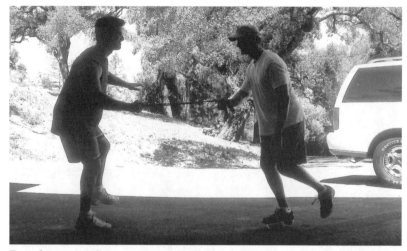 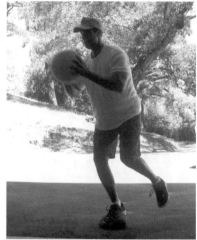

Tug-of-war standing on one leg on half a foam roll. *Keep a slight bend in your knees and relaxed ankles; stabilize your pelvis and spine while being tugged. The rule: You can't let go of the rope.*

Standing on a dyna-disc with one leg while throwing a medicine ball. *Keep a slight bend in your knees and relaxed ankles; minimize upper-body movement; stabilize your pelvis and spine.*

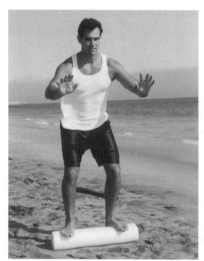 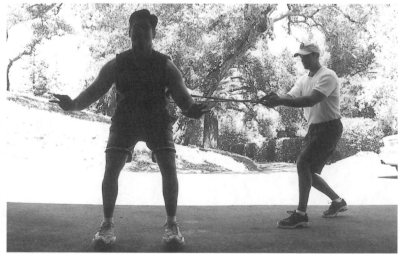

Standing on a full foam roll. *Maintain an athletic stance and neutral feet; keep your knees tracking over your second toes; upper-body movement should be minimal.*

Standing on half foam rolls while being pulled by a sport cord, eyes closed. *Maintain an athletic stance and relaxed ankles; stabilize your pelvis and spine while being pulled; keep your knees tracking over your second toes.*

Advanced Dynamic Balance Exercises

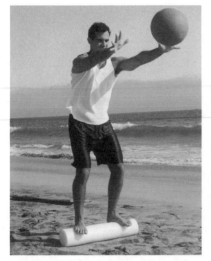

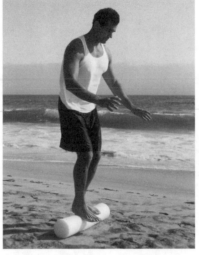

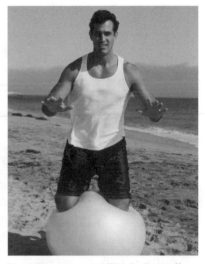

Standing on a full foam roll while tossing a medicine ball. *Maintain an athletic stance and neutral feet; keep your knees tracking over your second toes; toss and catch; stabilize your pelvis and spine.*

Log-rolling a full foam roll forward and backward. *Maintain neutral feet and minimal upper-body movement; keep your knees tracking over your second toes; take small steps.*

Kneeling on a stability ball. *Roll onto the ball using your hands; keep your knees apart, hips up, hands in front; stabilize your spine and pelvis.*

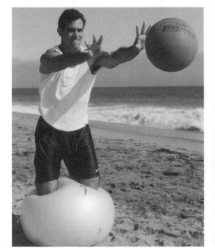

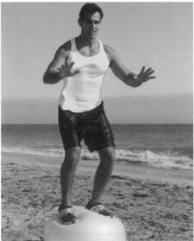

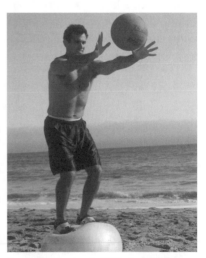

Kneeling on a stability ball while tossing a medicine ball. *Keep your knees apart, hips up, hands in front; toss and catch; stabilize your spine and pelvis; focus your eyes on a point in front of you.*

Standing on a stability ball. *Put the ball on a soft surface and have someone spot you. Mount the ball slowly. Maintain an athletic stance and look ahead, with your hands forward.*

Standing on a stability ball while tossing a medicine ball. *Put the ball on a soft surface and have a spotter. Maintain an athletic stance and look ahead, with hands forward; stabilize spine and pelvis.*

Advanced Dynamic Balance Exercises (continued)

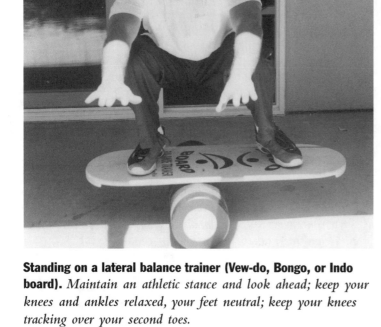

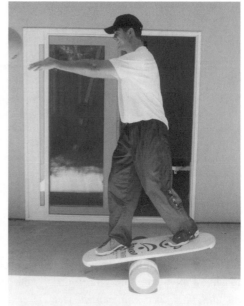

Standing on a lateral balance trainer (Vew-do, Bongo, or Indo board). *Maintain an athletic stance and look ahead; keep your knees and ankles relaxed, your feet neutral; keep your knees tracking over your second toes.*

Standing on a lateral balance trainer while tossing a medicine ball. *Maintain an athletic stance and look ahead; keep your knees and ankles relaxed, your feet neutral; toss and catch the ball; stabilize your spine and pelvis.*

on a stability ball is a great exercise to improve the strength and stability of your ankles, knees, hips, and trunk. Moreover, when this becomes easy, you can take it to another level by holding a medicine ball or wearing a weighted vest. This is the ultimate in sport-specific training and is essential for any elite athlete in a dynamic balance sport such as surfing.

Variety

It's important to have a lot of variety in the types of balance exercises you perform. As with anything, the body—and more specifically the nerv-

ous system—will adapt to a particular movement or direction of instability. In order to progress, you must instead constantly challenge your ability to balance dynamically with new and more difficult exercises. You'll find that once you've done an exercise for a while, your body will adapt, becoming very efficient and quickly making the adjustments necessary to keep you centered. If you continuously vary the exercises slightly and introduce more instability, you'll not only make bigger improvements in your ability to dynamically stabilize but also keep the workouts fun and do them more often!

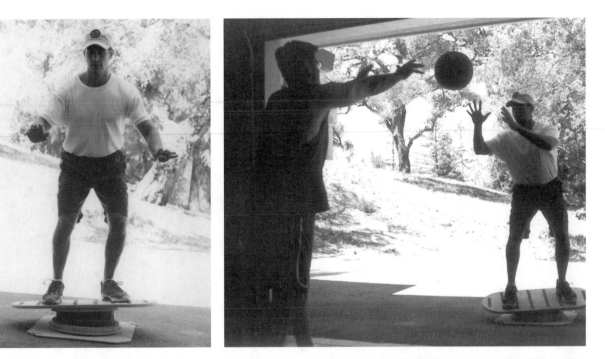

Standing on a rotating balance trainer that challenges lateral and fore–aft stability. *Maintain an athletic stance, minimal upper-body movement, and soft ankles and knees; stabilize your trunk.*

Standing on a rotating trainer that challenges lateral and fore–aft stability while tossing a medicine ball. *Maintain an athletic stance and minimal upper-body movement; toss and catch the ball; stabilize your trunk; look ahead.*

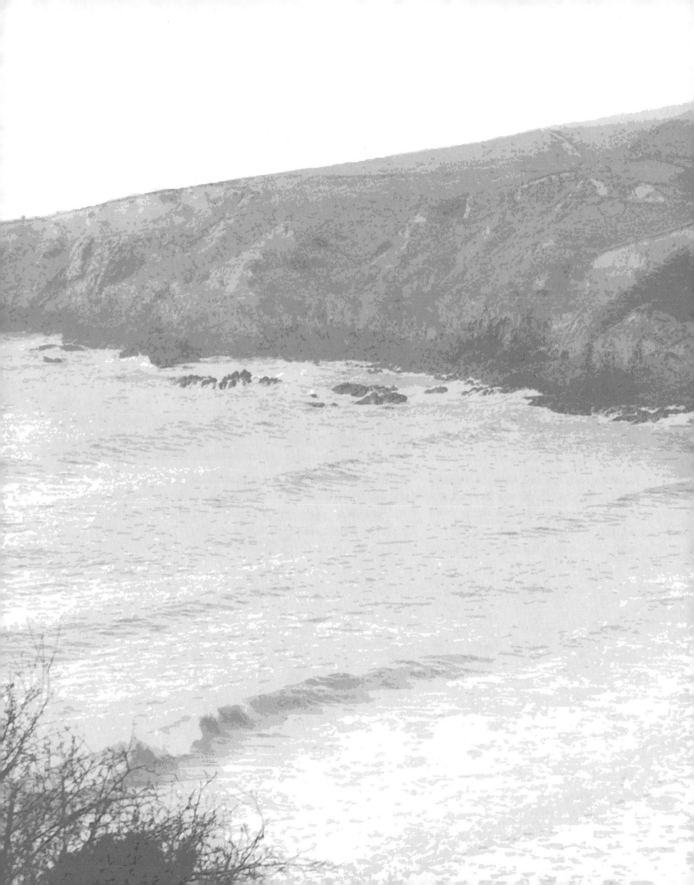

Chapter 11

HARD CORE Trunk Stabilization

You can't shoot a cannon from a canoe.

—Paul Chek, MSS, HHP, NMT, on the importance of core strength in athletics

Dynamic balance sports such as surfing require a high degree of *trunk stability*, or the ability to coordinate abdominal and back musculature and maintain an optimal spine and pelvis position during movement. By being able to stabilize the spine and pelvis, you accomplish three main things.

First, trunk stability protects the spine from trauma. Holding the spine in a biomechanically advantageous position and activating abdominal and back musculature during movement can prevent a variety of rotational and impact injuries to your spine and help keep your back healthy for life.

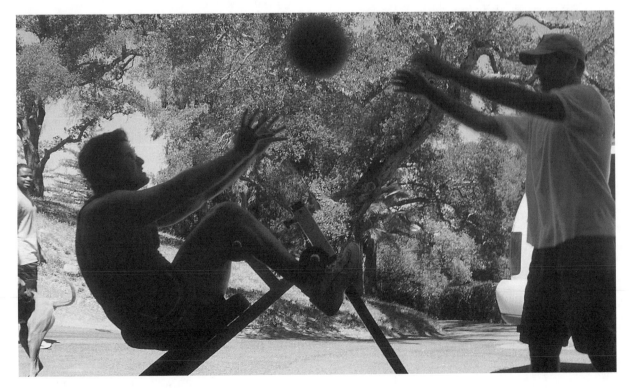

Using the core.

Second, as mentioned previously, trunk stability improves balance. Balance is enhanced by joint stability. The better you can stabilize every joint in your body, the better you'll be able to control movement. Human center of gravity or mass is slightly below and behind the navel. Thus, the better you can stabilize that point, the more effectively you can make subtle balance adjustments in your extremities.

Third, trunk stability increases strength and power. It's necessary to provide a solid platform from which the muscles of the extremities can then maximize their strength and power. The more complex or powerful the movement, the more important trunk stability becomes.

Stability of the trunk is dependent on core strength. There are many ways to strengthen the abdominal and back musculature, including popular exercises like "crunches." Such exercises,

however, recruit only very specific musculature. It's imperative to go one step further by performing movements that simultaneously strengthen multiple core stabilizers in order to maximize trunk strength and stability.

Anatomy of the Trunk

The most important trunk muscles are the *transverse abdominis* (the innermost abdominal wall), the *internal* and *external obliques* (the side abdominals), the *rectus abdominis* (the large outer muscles of the abdomen), the *latissimus dorsi* (the large back musculature), and the *erector spinae* (the smaller back musculature). Optimal strength, power, and balance require that these muscles work together in order to stabilize the core.

Neutral Spine

The term *neutral spine* refers to the position in which all the vertebrae are level in relation to one another. The spine runs from your head to your pelvis and has a natural curvature. There are three major portions: The cervical spine is essentially your neck, the thoracic portion is where your ribs attach, and the lumbar section is the lower back. The spine curves toward the rear of the body in the upper back and curves forward at the lumbar region. When it's in this neutral position, it is best able to disperse loads, provide a strong foundation for movement, and place the least amount of pressure on vertebral discs. The vertebral discs are made of soft tissue and act as mini shock absorbers in the back. If you're not in a neutral spine position, the vertebrae may be squeezing a disc, making it more prone to injury during movement. As a result, it's important to learn how to find and maintain this neutral spine position when you sit, walk, run, surf, and per-

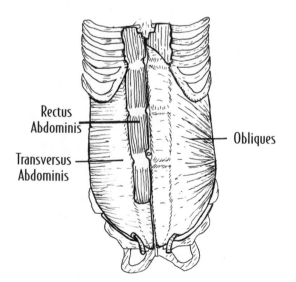

Rectus Abdominis

Transversus Abdominis

Obliques

The anterior abdominal wall, also known as the core.

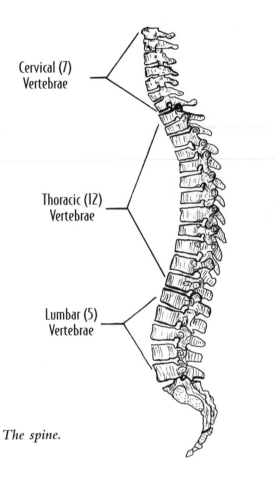

Cervical (7)
Vertebrae

Thoracic (12)
Vertebrae

Lumbar (5)
Vertebrae

The spine.

form any movement that may involve loading or rotation of the spine.

Many of us have developed poor postural habits and positions over the years that our tendons, ligaments, and muscles have become accustomed to. Breaking such habits may take a great deal of work, both stretching muscles that are tight (usually the chest musculature) and strengthening muscles that are weaker (generally the muscles of the back). Little did your parents know that reminding you not to slouch would not only make you look more respectable but also make you a better surfer!

Transverse Abdominis

The transverse abdominis (T.V.A.), for the majority of people, is the most neglected and detrained of the trunk musculature. As the inner abdominal wall, it can also be described as "the body's natural weight belt." This muscle connects to the thoraco-lumbar fascia of the back to form a ring around the core at the navel.

Merely learning how to activate the transverse abdominis can improve your trunk stability and balance immediately. The goal is that eventually, your body will become accustomed to contracting this "natural weight belt" prior to performing any movement.

Pulling the belly button in toward the spine can activate the transverse abdominis. This is not to be confused with sucking in your gut. Activation of the T.V.A. should result in a narrowing around the entire waist and a downward slope from the sternum or breastbone to the navel. Through training and awareness, everyone can learn to coordinate the contraction of the T.V.A. with every movement. At first, drawing the navel in before performing an exercise might feel awkward and difficult. Within a short period of time, though, it will become both comfortable and habitual. It's possible to continue to breathe normally and deeply despite drawing the navel in. Still, breaths are fuller in the mid-thoracic region and will feel increasingly more natural through practice.

Learning How to Activate the T.V.A.

One of the easiest ways to learn how to activate the T.V.A. is through the recruitment of the lower abdominal muscles. While lying faceup, with your knees bent and feet flat on the floor, place the ankle strap portion of your leash (or something similar) under the small of your back. Try to relax your entire body, especially your legs

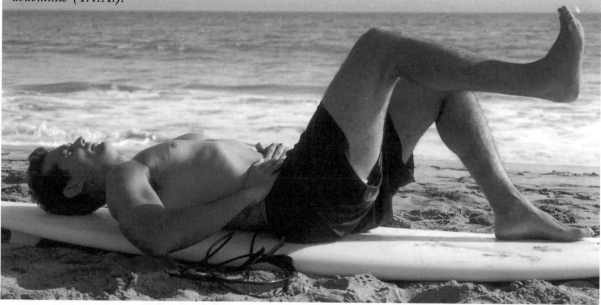

How to activate the transverse abdominis (T.V.A.).

and shoulders. Now draw in your navel, keeping one hand around your waist and the other on your belly. You should feel your midsection narrow and a downward slope from your chest to your hips. Next, alternate lifting each bent leg off the ground without losing pressure on the ankle strap, moving your pelvis, or affecting the downward slope and narrowed waist.

If your lower abdominals and/or T.V.A. are very weak, you'll find it difficult to keep your pelvis from moving when you lift your foot. In the event that the above exercise seems or becomes very easy, try it with a straight leg or with both legs bent simultaneously. Stellar lower abdominal strength and transverse activation would be to lower both straight legs at the same time from ninety degrees to the floor and up again without allowing your lower back to arch.

Trunk Strength and Stabilization Exercises

Some examples of surfing-specific core conditioning exercises appear on the following pages.

All trunk strength and stability movements should be done cautiously, with a neutral spine position and by first activating the transverse abdominis. You need a high level of T.V.A. awareness and strength—even during the easiest exercises—to protect your lower back. Most movements should be performed in a slow and controlled manner unless otherwise specified. It's best to perform the bulk of your core work at the end of your workout so these muscles are able to ast as effective stabilizers during other exercises. Also, be sure *not* to work muscles beyond the point of fatigue when you're most prone to injury. I also recommend that all exercises be done on a soft surface, in an open area, and with a spotter used for safety.

Hard Core for Life

Maintaining a strong and stable trunk not only will enhance your surfing performance but is in fact essential to staying active for life. The last thing you want to do is be sidelined from doing what you enjoy by chronic back pain!

Lower Rectus Abdominis Exercises Strong lower abs protect the lower back from injury.

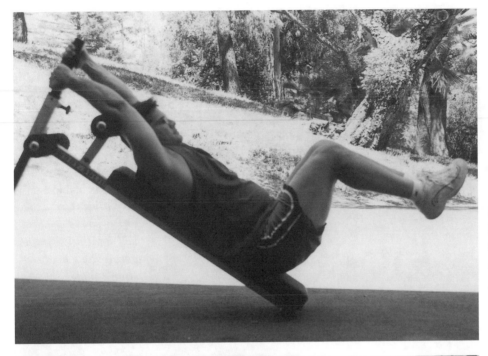

Relatively Easy
Lower abdominal leg curls off the bench. *Bring your knees to your chest. Your range of motion is limited by your ability to keep a neutral spine.*

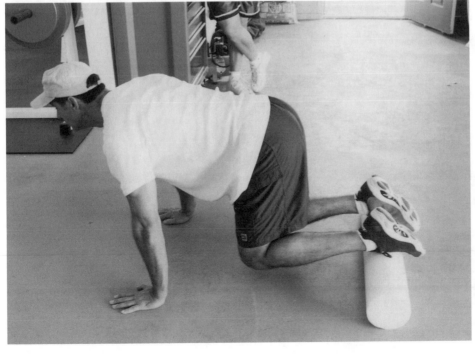

Advanced
Lower abdominal roll-outs on a foam roll. *Start with knees bent, hips level, and elbows slightly bent. Extend your legs.*

Lower Rectus Abdominis Exercises (continued)

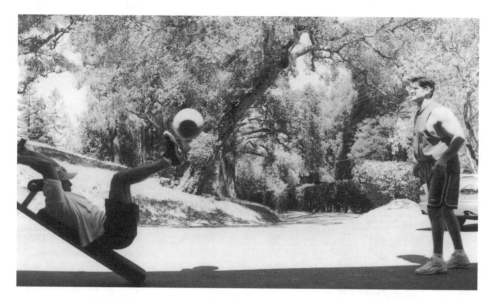

Very Advanced/Power Medicine ball kicks. *Explosive. Use a five- to ten-pound medicine ball and kick it to a partner. You need strong ankles.*

Oblique Exercises   Obliques facilitate upper-body rotation.

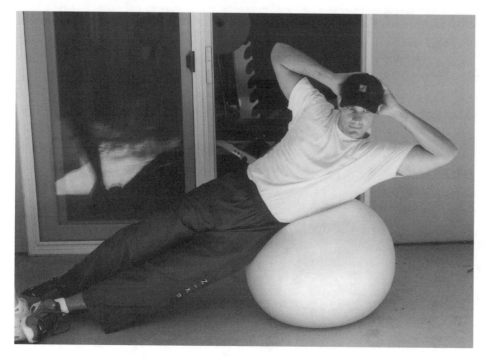

Relatively Easy Side crunches on a stability ball. *Keep your shoulders, hips, and knees in line, your inside leg forward.*

Oblique Exercises (continued)

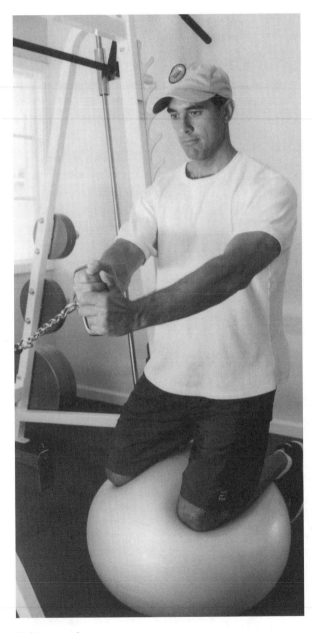

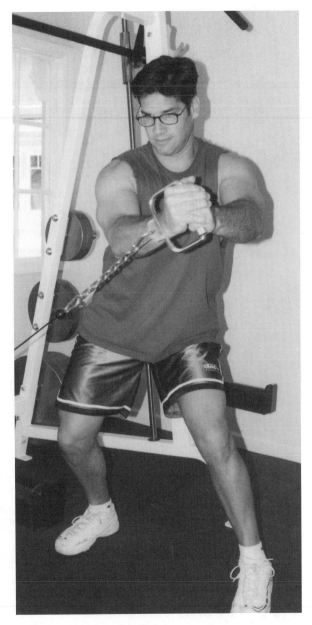

Advanced
Oblique cable pulls while kneeling on a ball. *Use light weight; keep your arms straight out in front and your trapezius relaxed as you pull the cable.*

Very Advanced/Power
Explosive standing cable pulls. *Powerful. Use medium weight; keep your arms straight; relax your trapezius. Pull the cable out fast; return slowly.*

Upper Rectus Abdominis Exercises Upper abs facilitate upper-body flexion.

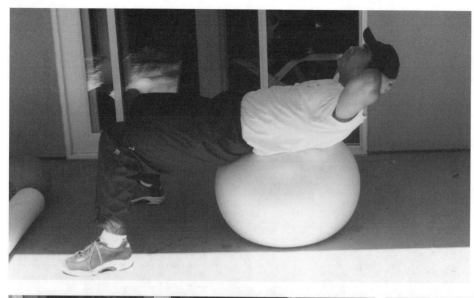

Relatively Easy
Crunches over a stability ball. *Look up. Keep your chin up; attempt to maintain a neutral spine by avoiding excessive flexion of the spine.*

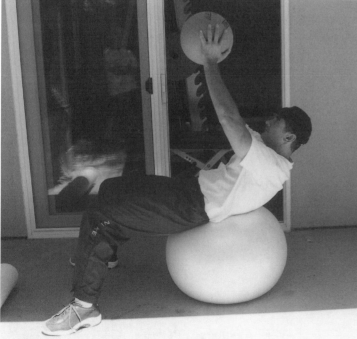

Advanced
Medicine ball crunches over a stability ball. *Hold a medium ball above your head; look up; avoid flexion.*

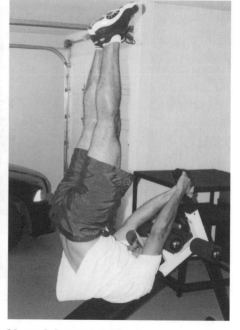

Very Advanced/Power
Pike-ups on a decline bench. *Explosive. Keep your knees bent as you go up; straighten your legs at the top; go down slowly.*

Erector Spinae Exercises The erector spinae facilitate upper-body extension.

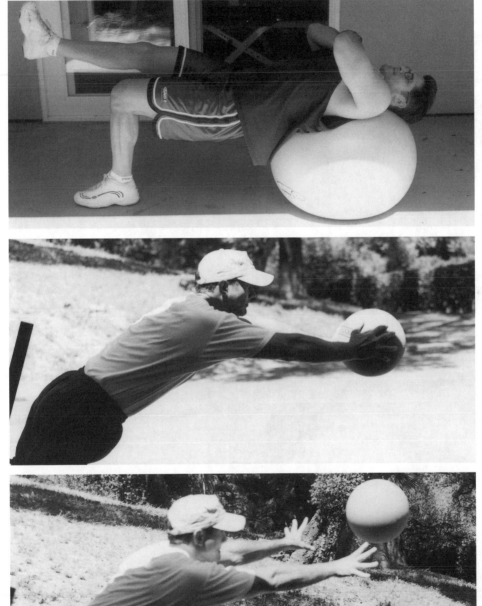

Relatively Easy
Bridge on a ball with alternate leg kicks. *Keep your shoulders on the ball, your gluts tight, and your pelvis level and up when you kick.*

Advanced
Back extensions while holding a medicine ball. *Your range of motion is limited by a neutral spine. Relax your trapezius.*

Very Advanced/Power
Back extensions while throwing a medicine ball. *Powerfully up, slowly down. Throw at the top, wait for the ball, then descend.*

Latissimus Dorsi Exercises   Lats assist in trunk stability as well as pulling movements, such as paddling.

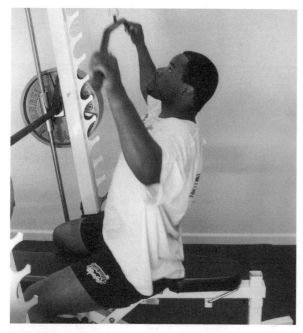

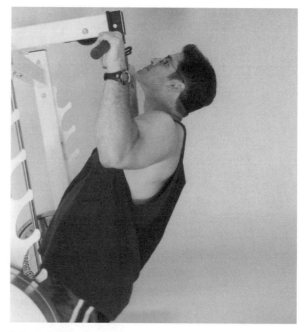

Relatively Easy
Front lat pull-downs. *At a slight angle, relax your traps, pull down keeping the bar in front, and squeeze your shoulder blades together.*

Advanced
Pull-ups. *Use a wide grip with palms down; relax your traps; pull up and avoid swinging; return slowly.*

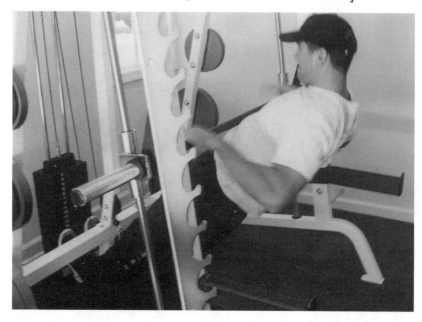

Very Advanced/Power
Explosive lat pulls from forty-five degrees. *Use a fixed bar; keep your body at forty-five degrees. Pull up explosively; return slowly.*

Overall Trunk Stability Exercises These exercises integrate a variety of trunk stabilizers.

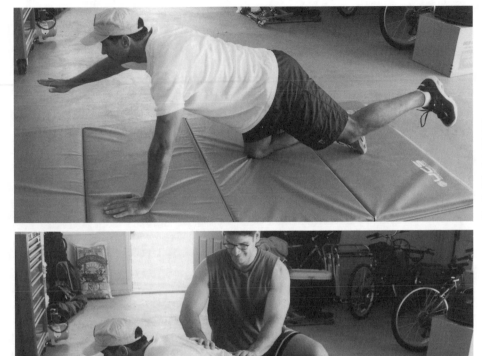

Relatively Easy
Dynamic quadruped.
Alternate extending your opposite leg and arm; keep hips and shoulders level.

Advanced
Quadruped stance partner challenge.
Extend your opposite leg and arm; close your eyes. Your partner will challenge your stability.

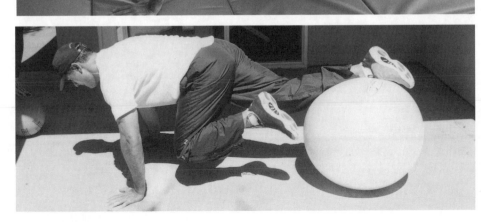

Very Advanced/Power
Stability ball sprinter pops. *Powerful. Maintain level hips and shoulders; alternate your legs; don't move the ball.*

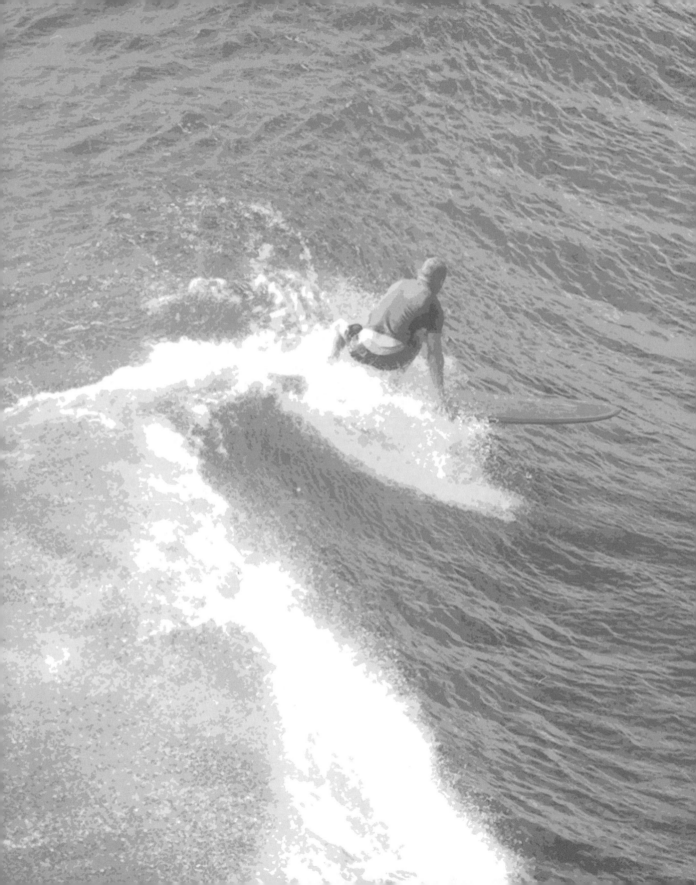

Chapter 12

RIPPED Strength Development

That which does not kill you, makes you stronger. —*Friedrich Nietzsche*

For decades, athletes and coaches in a variety of sports such as baseball, tennis, golf, basketball, and surfing rejected the idea of strength training. In fact, many dismissed the need for any type of cross-training. We now know, that athletes in every sport can enhance their performance by improving sport-specific fitness, balance, agility, quickness, speed, power, and strength through individualized cross-training workouts.

It's widely accepted that attempting to gain fitness by performing only your specific sport, for hours on end, can lead to fatigue that results in overuse injuries, unwanted biomechanical habits, and mental burnout. As you become fatigued, you are unable to stabilize joints properly, which can in turn lead to chronic injuries such as tennis elbow, runner's knee, jumper's knee, and numerous other nagging ailments. In skill sports such as tennis, golf, skiing, and surfing, it's common to also see a decrease in performance when athletes try to condition themselves by practicing their sport for several hours at a time. This is because as the primary musculature you use in your sport gets tired, you'll begin to recruit other muscles or adopt unusual body positions in order to compensate. The real killer is that it takes considerably more repetitions to correct a faulty movement pattern than it did to learn the movement the first time! Finally, variety is key to staying sharp not only physically but also mentally. Athletes without

diversity in their training programs burn out much more quickly than those who cross-train.

The vast majority of athletes in all sports incorporate some type of strength and power training into their programs. In fact, more than 75 percent of professional surfers are reportedly working out. However, when you mention strength and power development to many people, they still think football or bodybuilding.

For surfing, bulking up excessively would obviously be non–sport specific—and probably counterproductive. Many of us just haven't been exposed to the ways to enhance surfing performance through strength and power training. The amount of weight that's lifted, the type of motion used, the tempo at which it's performed, and the number of sets and repetitions in the workout will all affect the time that a muscle is put under tension. Moreover, this time-under-tension relationship should be determined by the demands of the sport and the goals of the athlete.

As we know, the demands of surfing are tremendous. Not only is it a ballistic or power sport, but if you surf daily, you're also exposing muscles, joints, and connective tissue to a great deal of stress. From a contest perspective, it's clear that the level of competition will only continue to improve. The success of those who don't currently train is achieved *in spite of*—not because of—having no customized, sport-specific program. As

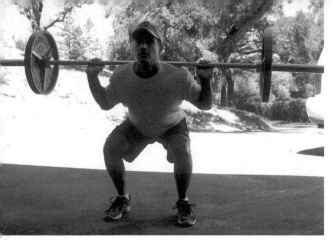

Strength.

surfing progresses, however, those who rely on talent alone will win fewer and fewer contests.

Sport Specificity

The sport of surfing requires a great deal of both strength and power. As we've discussed, a high strength-to-weight ratio must be developed in order to achieve efficient muscle movement. A surfer who can lift 300 pounds and weighs 150 is better off than a surfer who can lift 400 pounds but weighs 250. You must be able to move your mass effectively to excel in this sport. Adding the element of speed to your strength can then develop power. Paddling out, catching waves, and making aggressive bottom turns are ballistic moves that require explosive power. Again, it's important to have a high power-to-weight ratio opposed to just being powerful. For example, you might be able to throw a tire 50 feet. If you have a vertical jump of only 8 inches, however, you probably don't have the power-to-weight ratio necessary to pop up quickly or perform a maneuver off the lip.

It's important to develop strength and power as required by surfing's specific demands. Upper-body strength is necessary to paddle in the ocean safely. Upper-body power is essential to catching waves easily and standing up quickly. Lower-body strength is necessary to carve a sweeping arc. Lower-body power will help you perform explosive maneuvers.

Proprioception

As I mentioned in chapter 10, on stability, a stable joint is less prone to injury and promotes balance and efficiency. Joints are supported by tendons, ligaments, and muscles of varying sizes, that work together in making small and gross adjustments, depending on the type of movement. For example, paddling requires joint stability of the wrists, elbows, shoulders, and spine. The soft tissues surrounding all these joints work in unison to produce a fluid, efficient, and powerful paddle stroke. And common injuries like medial collateral ligament (MCL) tears, strains of the knee, and ankle sprains could be avoided by improving lower-body flexibility as well as joint strength and stability.

An important part of joint stability has to do with the nervous system. We have mechanoreceptors in the body that tell us the position and movement of limbs. The signals the central nervous system receives from the numerous mechanoreceptors are referred to as proprioception. We can train proprioception by integrating an element of instability in our strength sessions. As a result, our workouts become more sport specific as we challenge both the musculature and nervous system to respond in a way that's similar to the demands of surfing. Combining balance training with resistance training improves not only strength but also joint and trunk stability. And by forcing the body to recruit more stabilizing musculature, we get a more effective and efficient workout.

As we know, surfing is a dynamic balance sport, and the strength and power we're developing will do us little good if we're unable to utilize them in an unstable environment. Thus it's a good idea to integrate some level of instability in our strength and power training. This will mean that we'll have to decrease the resistance in order to make the exercise more sport specific and increase the demands on the nervous system.

Strength Development

Strength or resistance training is essential for both the competitive and recreational surfer. It's important to develop full-body overall strength in order to be safe in the ocean and have more enjoyable surfing sessions. Building strength is the first step toward creating joint stability. Once you're strong and stable, you can concentrate on developing power.

Tempo, Sets, Reps, and Resistance

As I mentioned earlier, time under tension affects the load placed on a muscle. Tempo is the speed at which a movement is performed. The tempo at which you perform an exercise will be determined by the amount of resistance and the desired goal. For strength training, you can slow the tempo to overload the muscle; power training, on the other hand, requires a quick tempo in order to develop speed.

The sets and repetitions (reps) performed in a workout will also affect the load on the muscle. For example, two sets of fifteen reps at a medium weight and a slow tempo might be used to train muscle endurance, whereas three sets of eight reps at a heavy weight could be used to build muscle mass. For the most part, the number of sets and repetitions is less important than the tempo and resistance of the exercise.

Many times athletes will alternate muscle groups during a workout. This gives each muscle a chance to recover but still keeps your heart rate up—and gets you out of the gym a little more quickly, too.

You can customize your program to match your goals, needs, wants, and abilities. The sets, reps, tempo, and resistance are all factors that can change the intensity and intent of a workout. Just remember that the average surfer doesn't want to train like the average guy in the weight room. Be selective in terms of what exercises you choose to do and how you choose to do them. Working out should be designed to enhance performance, not kill time!

Strength Training Exercises

It bears repeating that you don't want any increase in muscle mass to decrease your flexibility or range of motion. Therefore, every strength and power session should start with at least five minutes of aerobic warm-up and five to fifteen minutes of stretching; it should end with a cooldown and a ten- to twenty-minute stretch. This will help prevent injuries while you're working out as well as keep you from turning into a stiff-jointed musclehead!

What follows are some exercises that can help enhance surfing performance. Keep the resistance of each movement low when you're first starting out. It does little good to increase the weight of an exercise at the expense of form and technique. The goal is to not only make gains in strength and power but also train the body in correct or sport-specific biomechanical positions. The last thing you want is to create bad habits in the gym that could lead to injury or hurt the way you surf!

Variety

Just as we recognize the importance of incorporating variety in our balance training, we must continually challenge the nervous system in our strength training. This means varying the type of exercise, the angle it's performed at, the amount of stability, the resistance, the number of sets and reps, as well as the tempo. As a result, our bodies are forced continually to adapt, which will help us maximize our gains while decreasing monotony!

Upper-Body Strength Exercises

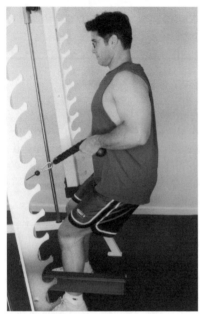

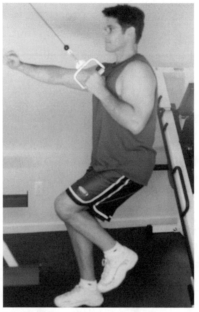

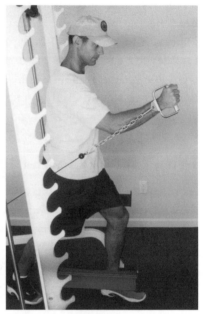

Latissimus Dorsi (Back)
Standing cable row. *Bend your knees, relax your traps, and squeeze your shoulder blades together.*

Latissimus Dorsi (Back)
Single-arm/single-leg cable pull. *Stand on the opposite leg with your knee slightly bent; relax your traps and stabilize your pelvis.*

Pectorals (Chest)
Single-arm cable chest press. *Use a staggered stance with your chest up. Relax your traps; pull the cable in front of your shoulders.*

Pectorals (Chest)
Dumbbell bench press on stability ball. *Stabilize your pelvis, squeeze your gluts, keep your hips up, and bend your arms to ninety degrees at the bottom.*

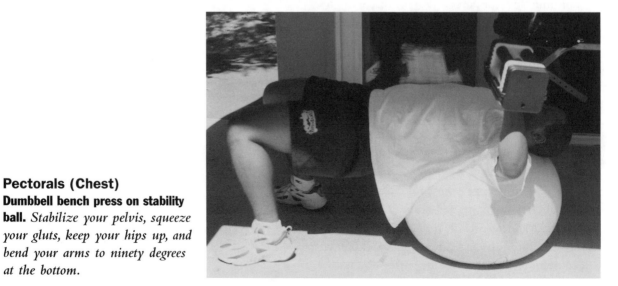

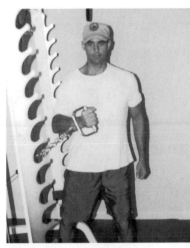

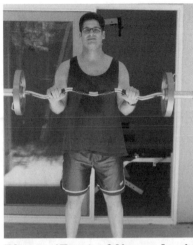

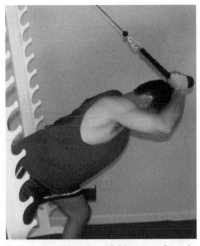

Deltoids (Shoulder)
Shoulder internal/external rotation.
Pull in for internal rotation, out for external. Stabilize your wrists; squeeze a towel with your elbow; use light resistance to maximize your range of motion.

Biceps (Front of Upper Arm)
Reverse arm curl. *Stabilize your wrists; keep your elbows to your sides; focus on your biceps and forearms as you lift; relax your traps.*

Triceps (Back of Upper Arm)
Standing tricep extension.
Stabilize your spine. Use a staggered stance. Start with your arms bent at ninety degrees, then extend them fully.

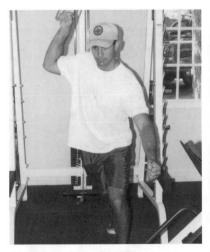

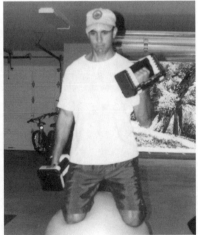

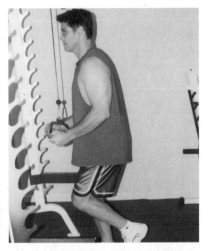

Deltoids (Shoulder)
Single-arm shoulder cable pull-down. *Stabilize your spine; use perfect posture; bring your shoulder up to ninety degrees and pull toward the floor.*

Biceps (Front of Upper Arm)
Dumbbell arm curl kneeling on a stability ball. *Stabilize your core, relax your traps, and alternate your arms; keep your chest up.*

Triceps (Back of Upper Arm)
Single-arm/single-leg cable tricep pull-down. *Standing on your opposite leg with your knee bent, stabilize your trunk. Start at nipple level with stable wrists and your palm facing up.*

Lower-Body Strength Exercises

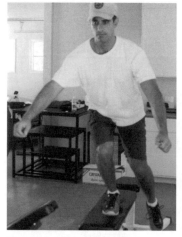

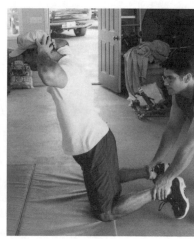

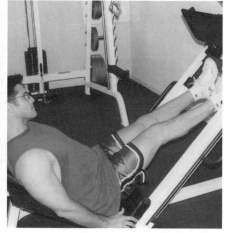

Quadriceps (Thighs)
Single-leg bench dip. *Level your hips and shoulders; keep your chest up, your feet neutral, and your knee over your second toe; bend to ninety degrees.*

Rectus Femoris (Hamstrings)
Eccentric hamstring. *Anchor your feet and lower toward the ground slowly. Push back up with your arms. Do not bend at the waist.*

Gastrocnemius and Soleus (Calves)
Calf raise on leg press machine. *With your toes on the end of the leg press plate, let your heels drop fully and extend onto the balls of your feet.*

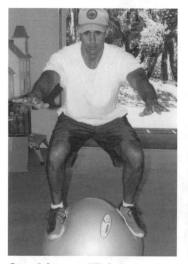

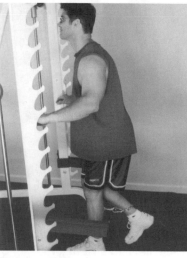

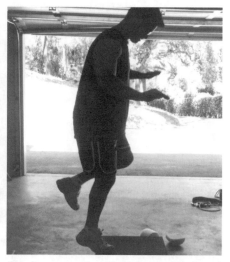

Quadriceps (Thighs)
Squats on a stability ball. *Stabilize your trunk; look ahead; bend to ninety degrees. Work in a safe area with a spotter.*

Rectus Femoris (Hamstrings)
Single-leg standing cable leg curl. *Stabilize your trunk and maintain a slight bend in your knee. Drag your toe on the ground.*

Gastrocnemius & Soleus (Calves)
Standing single-leg calf raise. *Stabilize your core; keep a slight bend in your knee; look ahead. Drop your heel and extend fully onto the ball of your foot.*

Chapter 13

BALLISTIC Power Development

Power training is to be done at 100% intensity at all times. If not done at this level, it is a waste of training time. —*The National Strength and Conditioning Association*

Explosive power is essential for both the competitive and recreational surfer. Surfing is a ballistic sport and requires quick, powerful movements. If we can train the body to adapt quickly to greater physical demands than what's required during our surf sessions, then we can enhance our explosive power. It's important to note that before we can develop power, we need a solid strength base in order to prevent injury and maximize explosiveness. Respect the progression and resist the urge to jump ahead. Safe and effective power training requires strong and stable joints. Improving power requires adaptations by our muscles, connective tissues, nervous systems, and energy systems. As a result, they all need to be prepared gradually for explosive movements. The first step is to build an adequate aerobic, agility, anaerobic, flexibility, joint stability, strength, and trunk stability base. We can then progress from the most basic power exercises to those that are higher impact.

Explosiveness

Explosiveness or *power* can be defined as your ability to exert maximal force as quickly as possible. In other words, strength plus speed equals power. It's possible to be strong and slow, or

weak and quick, and not powerful. In surfing, we may use our explosive power to catch a wave, pop up, arc a turn, or launch off the lip. In essence, we want to be as strong and as fast as we can for our body weight. It's all about power-to-weight ratio. Those who can move their mass the quickest and produce the most force will undoubtedly surf the most powerfully.

Sport Specificity

As I mentioned when discussing strength development, we want to train with our sport in mind. This means that we need to look at the forces involved in surfing to determine how we can best prepare for those demands. Both surfing and football require athletes to be powerful, for example. But since surfing shouldn't be a contact sport, we'll probably want to take a different approach to developing explosiveness. In any physical activity, athletes should analyze the cost-to-benefit ratio of what they do. In other words, what will we gain from training a particular way and what are the potential risks? I don't recommend that surfers go out and learn Olympic-type power lifts with heavy weight, for instance; although these can be great for athletes in some sports, the cost of performing such a lift with imperfect technique outweighs its possible bene-fits to us as surfers.

Tempo, Sets, Reps, and Resistance

As with strength training, the way you train to improve power is vital. The tempo should always be quick, since you're attempting to marry strength and speed. The sets and reps should be low in order to ensure that each effort is at maxi-mal intensity and to prevent overuse injuries. The resistance you use in your workouts should be rel-atively light. You don't want to sacrifice speed for the sake of loading up the weight. In fact, your body weight can serve as more-than-sufficient resistance for a multitude of power exercises.

Power Training Exercises

The best way to improve explosive power is through *plyometric training*—quick, powerful movements involving an eccentric contraction followed immediately by an explosive concentric contraction.

Jumping is an example of lower-body plyo-metrics. When you jump, you take off and land. The takeoff involves a concentric contraction of your muscles to accelerate your body weight. Upon landing, your muscles contract eccentri-cally in order to help you decelerate. Through training we can shorten the time between the two contractions to become more explosive. Throwing and catching a medicine ball with someone, or against a wall or trampoline, would be an example of upper-body plyometrics.

There are numerous plyometric exercises that are ideal for surfers. As with your agility workouts, I urge you to think critically, be cre-ative, stay safe, think sport specifically, and above all have fun!

The following are some guidelines for plyo-metric training.

- *Drills affecting a particular muscle or joint should not be performed two days in a row.* This is necessary to allow muscles, ligaments, and tendons adequate recovery time and pre-vent injury.
- *Allow time for complete recovery between sets.* Because power training should be done at 100 percent intensity, you need to let your heart rate and respirations come down between efforts.
- *Use footwear and landing surfaces that offer good shock absorption.* This will help mini-mize impact and prevent injury.
- *Warm up thoroughly and stretch before per-forming any plyometric exercises.* This will prepare muscles, ligaments, and tendons for the strenuous exercise they'll be doing and help prevent injury.
- *As the stress level of the movement increases, so too should the complexity.* In other words, as an exercise becomes easy, keep your nervous system challenged by incorporating direction changes, requiring more accuracy, or involving a medicine ball.
- *Proper technique is essential and should never be sacrificed.* As technique declines, the risk of injury increases tremendously.
- *The time spent in contact with the floor or medicine ball should be as short as possible.* Decreasing contact time results in an increase in speed, which will ultimately improve power.
- *The time spent in contact with the floor or medicine ball should be as quiet as possible.* When you're quiet, you're training muscles to utilize just the right amount of eccentric con-

traction to decelerate your body weight or the ball, which will enhance speed and prevent injury.

- *Make sure your spine and pelvis are stabilized by your trunk musculature at all times.* This will help you maintain control over your center of mass and minimize the forces incurred by your spine.
- *Be aware of posture and body positions during all drills.* To keep your plyometric training sport specific, train your body to be powerful—but not at the expense of control.

Variety

Because power training involves adaptations by the nervous system as well as muscles and connective tissue, it's imperative that we make an effort to vary our exercises. Once our nervous systems adjust to the physical demands we're placing on them, we need to add more stress and complexity to our exercises in order to achieve the most benefit. Variety keeps us challenged and will eventually yield the greatest results. If we continually up the ante in all aspects of our surfing preparation, we can expand our comfort zone and in turn enhance our performance.

Upper-Body Power Exercises

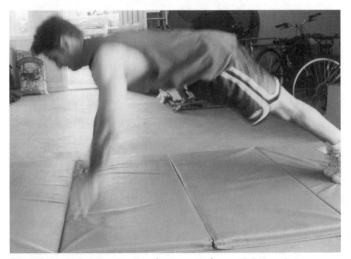

Clapping push-up. *An explosive push-up. Maintain a neutral spine, clap while in the air, and land with bent arms.*

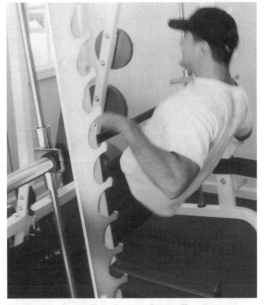

Explosive forty-five-degree lat pull. *Start at forty-five degrees from the bar; relax your traps; pull your chest toward the bar quickly.*

Lower-Body Power Exercises

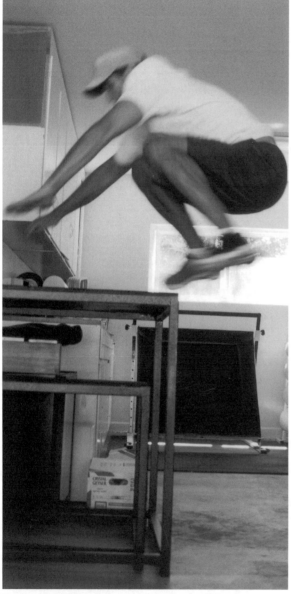

Vertical jump onto box. *With feet and knees at shoulder width, jump explosively. Land softly, flexing your knees and ankles fully.*

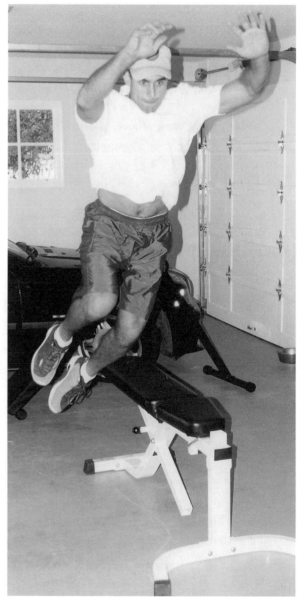

Lateral jump over bench. *Level your shoulders and hips; look ahead. Make an explosive jump to the side with a soft landing.*

Chapter 14

THE GAME PLAN Designing a Training Program

Physical preparation is the very key to performance. It should not be left to happenstance and it should not be relegated to a "time filler" position in your program. —*Steve Johnson, Ph.D., sports science innovator*

By taking an interest in enhancing your surfing performance, you already possess one of the most essential attributes of a successful athlete: You are goal-oriented. You want to maximize your time, energy, and focus in order to realize the objective of surfing better. Well, the first step to success is to design a customized, functional, effective training program that takes into consideration your goals, needs, wants, and abilities. In other words, instead of surfing, running, swimming, or lifting only when you feel like it, sit down and create a training program for yourself that incorporates all the elements that you want to work on. For example, you'll want to spend more time swimming, running, and lifting in the off season than during the competition months. You'll also want to gradually increase the length and intensity of such workouts as your fitness improves. Since time and energy are limited resources, however, you'll need to cut back on certain workouts in order to concentrate on other types of training as the competitive season approaches. The idea is to devise a game plan for yourself that will incorporate all the aspects of surfing performance and give you the best chance of reaching your goals.

There are numerous factors that go into designing a training program. Two athletes could be the same age and have the same goal but will more than likely differ in terms of the amount of time they have available per week, skill level, strengths, weaknesses, motivation, dedication, overall fitness, and personality. As a result, a training program needs to be customized to each individual. It's misleading to make a blanket statement such as "everyone should do this," because you could very likely be the exception. My goal is to get people to start thinking more critically about what they're doing. Although there may be one training program that will work adequately for a great deal of average surfers, I don't want to promote mediocrity. I want to empower you by intelligently educating you on what's out there, in the hope that you can eventually build something to take you to the next level.

Periodization

The term *periodization* refers to the way the volume and intensity of your workouts are cycled from day to day, week to week, month to month, and even year to year in a training program. A microcycle is usually a seven-day block of training, or one week. A macrocycle can consist of four, six, or even eight microcycles. Putting together multiple macrocycles with the same overall intent is referred to as a phase of training; multiple phases are called a period. Finally, each year or season is usually broken up into at least two periods that can last anywhere from two weeks to several months. It's important to note that periodization doesn't mean that you perform only specific workouts during a particular phase of training, but rather that you are putting more emphasis on certain elements of your development.

For instance, I recommend dividing each year into a preparation period, competition period, and a prolonged active rest period. The preparation period starts with a general conditioning phase and becomes more surfing specific as you approach your contest months. Since contests are held throughout the year at various levels, this time frame could vary from year to year. The competition period should then build toward one or two peak macrocycles, when you want to be at your absolute best both physically and psychologically. If you're not a contest surfer, the competition period would simply be the winter or the time of year that you surf the most. Finally, the active rest period should last four to six weeks, and follows the competition period. I call it an active rest period because you don't sit on the couch all day, but simply take a break from structured training. This is a time to surf when you want, play some golf, and perhaps, if you feel like it, go for the occasional run, skate, or swim. In essence, the active rest period allows for much-needed recovery so that you can do it all over again!

Here's how a year of training might be designed:

Rest Period—Six Weeks

- Nothing structured or too strenuous.
- Your goal is to achieve complete physical and psychological recovery.

Preparation Period—Twenty-Six Weeks

- Overall fitness and conditioning phase—eight weeks.
- Strength, aerobic, and technique development phase—eight weeks.
- Power, anaerobic, and style development phase—eight weeks.
- Contest specialization phase—two weeks.

Competition Period—Twenty Weeks

- Three competition macrocycles—twelve weeks total.
- First peak macrocycle—four weeks.
- Second peak macrocycle—four weeks.

A macrocycle of training will become gradually more difficult from the first to third week and then relatively easy the fourth week. The third week of the program is the most challenging, and the fourth week is a recovery week. This recovery time is necessary in order for the body to make adaptations to the hard work it has done.

We refer to microcycles in terms of our intended volume and intensity for that week. A four-week macrocycle, for instance, should progress from a relatively low-intensity week to a medium, high, and finally a recovery microcycle. The week(s) we want to be at our best during the season is called a peak week, and the week right before that is referred to as a taper microcycle. It's difficult to peak more than one or two times per competition period. The overall volume and intensity of each microcycle in relation to the others in that macrocycle will ultimately affect your performance and needs to be carefully considered.

It's important to periodize your training throughout the week so that you can best manage your time and energy. Hard workouts such as power, strength, and interval training require a great deal of energy. If you go into these workouts fatigued, you'll accomplish far less than you could if you were well rested. Many athletes who don't periodize their training become flat or sluggish and are at a greater risk for injury and overtraining.

For instance, if you generally attend weekend contests, you'll want Monday and Friday to be your relatively easy days. I say *relatively* because depending on the overall volume and intensity of the week, you might take the day completely off or just take it easier in comparison to the other days that week. In this example, you'd want to schedule your most intense workouts on Tuesday and, if you don't have a contest, Saturday. You can then plan your higher-volume, lower-intensity workouts for Wednesday and, when there's no contest, Sunday. This leaves Thursday as a wild card day or a day you can dedicate to the specific surfing element you're trying to improve during that phase of your training.

Training Volume and Intensity within Each Macrocycle

Week 1	Relatively low volume and intensity
Week 2	Greater volume and intensity than week 1
Week 3	Greater volume and intensity than week 2
Week 4	Lower volume and intensity than week 1

Training Volume and Intensity within Each Week

Monday	Complete rest or active rest (short, easy run or balance/agility workout)
Tuesday	High intensity/low volume (intervals, power, strength)
Wednesday	High volume/low intensity (a long aerobic workout)
Thursday	Medium volume/medium intensity (should reflect goal of that phase of training)
Friday	Same as Monday
Saturday	Contest or same as Tuesday
Sunday	Contest or same as Wednesday

Competition-Period Macrocycle for an Experienced Contest Surfer

Microcycle 1 (Low Week)

DAY	ACTIVITY	TIME	INTENSITY	INTENT
Monday	Off			
Tuesday	Surf session	1½ hours	Medium	Technique/style
	Intervals	30 minutes	Medium	Improve A.T.
	Power	1 hour	High	Strength/power
	Stretch	15 minutes	Low	Flexibility
Wednesday	Surf session	1½ hours	Medium	Technique/style
	Rowing machine	20 minutes	Medium	Aerobic
	Run	25 minutes	Medium	Aerobic
	Stretch	15 minutes	Low	Flexibility
Thursday	Surf session	1½ hours	Medium	Technique/style
	Strength	30 minutes	Medium	Strength/stability
	Core strength	15 minutes	Medium	Trunk stability
	Stretch	15 minutes	Low	Flexibility
Friday	Surf session	1 hour	Low	Fun/relax
	Balance/agility	30 minutes	Medium	Stability/speed
	Stretch	15 minutes	Low	Flexibility
Saturday	Surf session	1½ hours	High	Simulate contest
	Strength	45 minutes	Medium	Strength
	Core strength	15 minutes	Medium	Trunk stability
	Stretch	15 minutes	Low	Flexibility
Sunday	Surf session	2 hours	High	Simulate contest
	Run on beach	30 minutes	Low	Aerobic
	Stretch	15 minutes	Low	Flexibility

Competition-Period Macrocycle for an Experienced Contest Surfer

Microcycle 2 (Medium Week)

DAY	ACTIVITY	TIME	INTENSITY	INTENT
Monday	Off			
Tuesday	Surf session	1½ hours	Medium	Technique/style
	Intervals	30 minutes	Medium	Improve A.T.
	Power	1 hour	High	Strength/power
	Core strength	15 minutes	Medium	Trunk stability
	Stretch	15 minutes	Low	Flexibility
Wednesday	Surf session	2 hours	Medium	Technique/style
	Rowing machine	20 minutes	Medium	Aerobic
	Run	25 minutes	Medium	Aerobic
	Stretch	15 minutes	Low	Flexibility
Thursday	Surf session	1½ hours	Medium	Technique/style
	Strength	45 minutes	Medium	Strength/stability
	Core strength	15 minutes	Medium	Trunk stability
	Stretch	15 minutes	Low	Flexibility
Friday	Surf session	1½ hours	Low	Fun/relax
	Swim	30 minutes	Medium	Aerobic
	Stretch	15 minutes	Low	Flexibility
Saturday	Surf session	1½ hours	High	Simulate contest
	Balance/agility	25 minutes	Medium	Stability/speed
	Core strength	5 minutes	Medium	Trunk stability
	Stretch	15 minutes	Low	Flexibility
Sunday	Contest	2 hours	High	Competition
	Stretch	15 minutes	Low	Flexibility

Competition-Period Macrocycle for an Experienced Contest Surfer

Microcycle 3 (High Week)

DAY	ACTIVITY	TIME	INTENSITY	INTENT
Monday	Run on beach	30 minutes	Medium	Aerobic
	Stretch	15 minutes	Low	Flexibility
Tuesday	Surf session	1½ hours	Medium	Technique/style
	Intervals	45 minutes	High	Improve A.T.
	Power	1 hour	High	Strength/power
	Core strength	15 minutes	Medium	Trunk stability
	Stretch	15 minutes	Low	Flexibility
Wednesday	Surf session	2 hours	Medium	Technique/style
	Rowing machine	20 minutes	Medium	Aerobic
	Run	25 minutes	Medium	Aerobic
	Stretch	15 minutes	Low	Flexibility
Thursday	Surf session	1½ hours	Medium	Technique/style
	Strength	45 minutes	Medium	Strength/stability
	Core strength	15 minutes	Medium	Trunk stability
	Stretch	15 minutes	Low	Flexibility
Friday	Surf session	1½ hours	High	Simulate contest
	Balance/agility	25 minutes	Medium	Stability/speed
	Core strength	5 minutes	Medium	Trunk stability
	Stretch	15 minutes	Low	Flexibility
Saturday	Contest	2 hours	High	Competition
	Stretch	15 minutes	Low	Flexibility
Sunday	Contest	2 hours	High	Competition
	Stretch	15 minutes	Low	Flexibility

Competition-Period Macrocycle for an Experienced Contest Surfer

Microcycle 4 (Recovery Week)

DAY	ACTIVITY	TIME	INTENSITY	INTENT
Monday	Off			
Tuesday	Surf session	1½ hours	Medium	Technique/style
	Strength	30 minutes	Medium	Strength/stability
	Core strength	15 minutes	Medium	Trunk stability
	Stretch	15 minutes	Low	Flexibility
Wednesday	Surf session	1½ hours	Medium	Technique/style
	Swim	30 minutes	Medium	Aerobic
	Stretch	15 minutes	Low	Flexibility
Thursday	Surf session	1½ hours	Medium	Fun/relax
	Balance/agility	15 minutes	Medium	Stability/speed
	Stretch	15 minutes	Low	Flexibility
Friday	Off			
Saturday	Surf session	1½ hours	Medium	Technique/style
	Strength	30 minutes	Medium	Strength
	Core strength	15 minutes	Medium	Trunk stability
	Stretch	15 minutes	Low	Flexibility
Sunday	Surf session	1½ hours	Medium	Technique/style
	Stretch	15 minutes	Low	Flexibility

Be Realistic

Designing an effective training program can be a time-consuming process. As you gain more knowledge and experience of how to train, you'll become more proficient at developing the game plan that will suit you the best. The important thing is that you remain realistic. You need to be honest with yourself in assessing how much time you have each week to train, how much energy you have, and, most importantly, how committed you are to reaching your goals.

Follow Through

Once you've created a plan for getting where you want to go, stick with it as best you can. If you've taken into consideration your goals, needs, wants, and abilities, then every workout must have a purpose. To follow your program only sporadically will simply not be effective. Still, there will be times when you'll need to cut yourself some slack. If you get sick, for example, take it easy and make sure you're recovered. When you feel better, look at how you can ease your way back into your training program. Perspective is as important as dedication. You didn't get to your present level of fitness and skill in a week, and you definitely won't lose it in a week!

Reassess

I cannot stress the importance of this enough. You need to constantly reassess the effectiveness of what you're doing. I recommend keeping a training log of your workouts and periodically analyzing it to look for ways you can improve. Becoming a great surfer is a process. Over time, you'll observe patterns in your training that can help you tweak your game plan for the better. At the end of each year, you'll be able to take a step back and reevaluate your strengths, weaknesses, goals, likes, and dislikes to create an even more effective training program for the coming season!

Chapter 15

HEAD GAMES Sports Psychology and Surfing

As you think, you become. —*Thomas Edison*

In previous chapters, we've discussed in depth how surfing is a skill sport that requires a great deal of physical conditioning. Recently, the sport has increased in popularity both recreationally and competitively, bringing with it marketing dollars and sponsorship, which have in turn motivated athletes to seek a greater competitive edge. Typically, surfers are very independent and resist structure when pursuing their sport. It's becoming increasingly clear, however, that a mental game plan can be just as important at enhancing surfing performance as your physical game plan.

The six-time world champion surfer Kelly Slater was once quoted before a competition as saying, "This has nothing to do with anyone else but me. I have to make it simple—I have to know what the conditions are doing. I have to know when I take off on a wave; it's not a crappy wave. I have to take off on good waves and I have to surf them well. I have to get deep." Kelly's psychological approach—not being distracted by what others are doing, and focusing on the basics—makes it easier for him to consistently surf to his potential. Likewise, you need to develop your own optimal mental strategy. The essentials of such a plan involve developing ways to relax, concentrate, and image more effectively.

Relaxation

Relaxation strategies are critical as part of a surfer's mental game plan. It is common for big-wave surfers, for instance, to fear being held under water. This fear can lead to panic, and panic can kill. Big-wave surfer Ken Bradshaw was once quoted as saying, "I don't fear drowning, I fear panicking." Shallow-reef or rock-break surfing can also lead to serious injury. In competitive surfing, as in any sport, performance anxiety is common. Surfers are under pressure to score waves during timed heats against other surfers. They feel the pressure of having to outperform their competitors in front of judges. The muscular tension that results from the anxiety a surfer would feel in any of these situations can adversely affect athleticism and ultimately performance.

One example of a relaxation strategy for surfing is rhythmic breathing. This can easily be done before getting into the water or between wave sets. Breathing exercises have proven very effective in reducing anxiety. For instance, when you notice that you're feeling tension, take three to five deep, diaphragmatic breaths. Each breath consists of inhaling to a count of four, holding for a count of four, exhaling for a count of four, and pausing for a count of four before repeating the sequence.

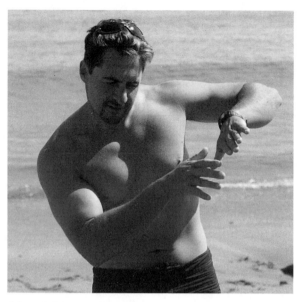

Mental imagery.

Concentration

Concentration strategies are also a crucial part of a surfer's mental game plan. Big-wave surfers can drown by being caught in the impact zone or missing a takeoff. A crowded surf area requires you to be cognizant of your position in relation to the waves *and* to those around you in order to be safe. Competitive surfers obviously need to be focused in order to perform complex maneuvers to their potential. These athletes encounter external distracters such as other surfers and announcement speakers. They also may be struggling with internal distractions such as negative self-talk or pessimistic thought processes.

One example of a concentration strategy you could try is attentional cuing. You can do this before getting into the water, between wave sets, or even between maneuvers on a wave. Attentional cues can be verbal or kinesthetic and are used to retrigger focus once it has been lost. These cues can help you center your attention

on the most appropriate aspects of the task at hand. For example, you might find it beneficial to concentrate on where your weight is during a top-turn maneuver. Your attentional cue might be "rear foot, outside rail." These four words might help you focus on the elements that are most critical to performing the skill well.

Imagery

Mental rehearsal strategies can also be very effective for surfers. Any athlete in the sport could benefit from rehearsing the selection of surfable waves, successful takeoffs, and enjoyable rides. Big-wave surfers can increase confidence by imagining a successful outcome. Truly big waves are rare, so when the waves are generally small, you can stay mentally prepared for what it will feel and look like to charge for a mountainous wall of water. Hesitation can be deadly in this situation. Competitive surfers can benefit from imagining heat strategy, the maneuvers they will perform, making critical sections of a wave, and surfing with a smooth, fluid style that the judges will like.

One effective mental rehearsal strategy is visualization, which you can work on anytime you're out of the water or between wave sets. Simply imagine all the elements of a successful performance in great detail, using as many senses as possible as you create the event in your mind. Once you're experienced at visualization, you might be able to actually smell the sea air and taste the salt water, for instance, during an imagery session.

Positive Self-Talk

Self-talk is what we tell ourselves or think about before, during, and after an event. In surfing, we can enhance performance by using positive self-talk in order to develop more confidence.

Identifying areas where we need more confidence and then creating some positive statements to say or write on a regular basis can help accomplish this. Here are some examples:

- I generate speed well when the waves are small.
- I always land big airs.
- I enjoy contests and surf well under pressure.

It's essential that any affirmation be stated strongly and in the present tense.

Athletes in countless sports have realized the benefits of replacing negative thoughts with positive ones. It does us no good to think about what we don't want to happen or things that are out of our control. In a way, our brain is like a computer. The better our instructions, the sweeter the results!

Precompetition Routine

For many athletes, contest day can be stressful. Besides the anxiety of wanting to do well, you're concerned with things such as making sure you have everything you need and are in the right place at the right time. A good way to manage the stress and help you stay organized is to develop a precompetition routine. This can be likened to a jet in autopilot mode. A routine will allow you to relax more and simplify your preparation on contest day, which will in turn help you focus on what's important.

Through experience, you'll be able to create a system for the optimal way to prepare for an event. For example, you might want to warm up and stretch a certain number of minutes before your first heat. And perhaps you'll get into a habit of getting away from everyone at some point so that you can relax, concentrate, and visualize what you're trying to accomplish. A lot of athletes also use music to get psyched up or calm nerves before competition.

Your precompetition routine might seem somewhat generic and forced at first, but over time you'll be able to customize and tweak it so that it becomes more comfortable. You may even decide that you perform best when there's little or no structure to what you do the day before and the day of a contest. Whatever your contest-day preparation includes, it should put you in a frame of mind that will lead to total domination!

Mental Cross-Training

Just as physical cross-training is crucial to your surfing, it's also important to cross-train mentally. For example, sports like golf can help you improve your ability to relax, concentrate, or visualize. Applying mental training strategies in a variety of situations will increase your awareness and understanding of the techniques while improving your ability to use them.

Training Logs

Athletes in most sports keep a log of the factors that can affect their performance. This is a great way to see patterns in your training or contests so that you can design a better program in the future. For example, if you notice that you usually aren't surfing well when the bigger events come along, you might be able to tweak your training to prevent this from happening in the future.

A good training log should allow you to keep track of any physical and psychological factors that you think might affect your surfing. Yet it also needs to be fairly easy to read and not too time consuming to fill out.

What follows is an example of a training log I developed for some of the surfers I've coached.

NAME: _____

Monday / /	Weather Conditions	Training Workout	Hours Planned	Comments
Hours of Sleep			Actual Hours	
Breakfast			Surf Conditions	
Lunch			Subjective Rating	
Dinner				

NAME: _____

Tuesday / /	Weather Conditions	Training Workout	Hours Planned	Comments
Hours of Sleep			**Actual Hours**	
Breakfast			**Surf Conditions**	
Lunch			**Subjective Rating**	
Dinner				

NAME: _____

Wednesday / /	Weather Conditions	Training Workout	Hours Planned	Comments
Hours of Sleep			Actual Hours	
Breakfast			Surf Conditions	
Lunch				
Dinner			Subjective Rating	

NAME: _____

Thursday / /	Weather Conditions	Training Workout	Hours Planned	Comments
Hours of Sleep			Actual Hours	
Breakfast			Surf Conditions	
Lunch				
Dinner			Subjective Rating	

NAME: _____

Friday / /	Weather Conditions	Training Workout	Hours Planned	Comments
Hours of Sleep			Actual Hours	
Breakfast			Surf Conditions	
Lunch				
Dinner			Subjective Rating	

NAME: _____

Saturday / /	Weather Conditions	Training Workout	Hours Planned	Comments
Hours of Sleep				
Breakfast			Actual Hours	
Lunch			Surf Conditions	
Dinner			Subjective Rating	

NAME: _____

Sunday / /	Weather Conditions	Training Workout	Hours Planned	Comments
Hours of Sleep				
			Actual Hours	
Breakfast				
			Surf Conditions	
Lunch				
			Subjective Rating	
Dinner				

Total Training Hours	Contest Results/ Notes	Comments on the Week	Goals for Next Week
Subjective Rating	**Learning Experiences**		

The End Result

As our sport increases in popularity, a growing number of us will focus on the mental aspects of our performance. It is clear that having a mental game plan can aid in achieving our potential. Relaxation, concentration, and imagery strategies can be extremely useful mental training tools. When combined with effective physical preparation, psychological preparation can mean the difference between disappointment and victory!

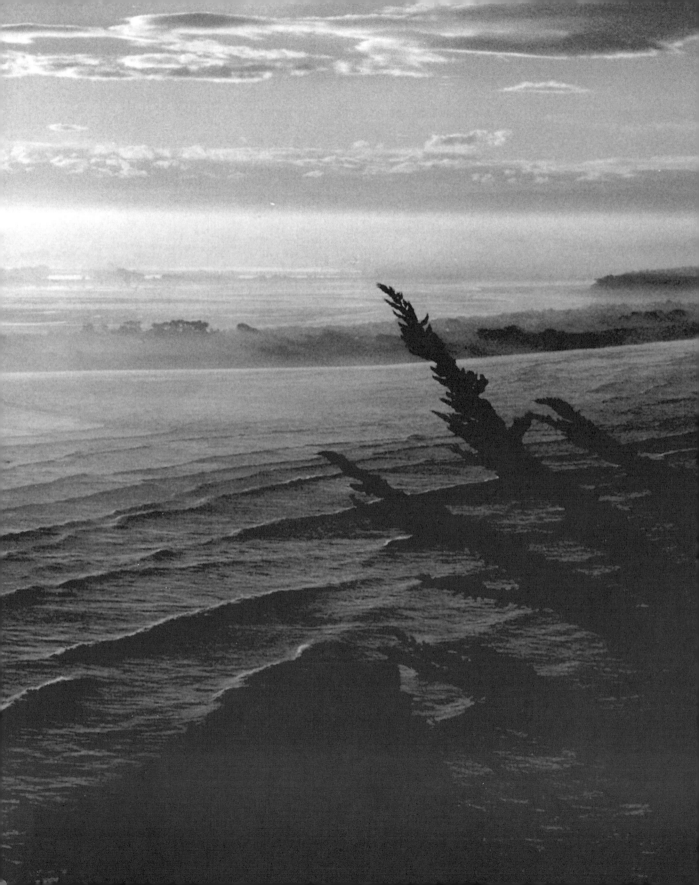

GLOSSARY OF SURF LINGO

Aerial: An advanced maneuver in which the board is launched off the lip of the wave at high speed.

Aerobic: Physical work in which the body is able to supply oxygen to meet the demands of working muscles; fat is the primary energy source.

Aerobic capacity: The ability to sustain a medium-intensity aerobic effort for extended periods of time.

Anaerobic: Physical work in which working muscles aren't getting an adequate supply of oxygen; glycogen is the primary energy source.

Anaerobic endurance: The ability to sustain a high-intensity anaerobic effort for short periods of time and recover fairly quickly between those efforts.

Anaerobic threshold: The point during exercise at which working muscles go into oxygen debt; the point at which fat is no longer used as an energy source.

Angling: Taking off at an angle away from the breaking part of the wave.

Arc: A term used in skiing, snowboarding, and surfing to describe the shape of a well-executed turn.

ASP: Association of Surfing Professionals.

Axed: When a surfer falls as a result of being hit by the breaking lip of the wave.

Backside: Surfing with your back to the wave.

Bailing: Diving off the surfboard, usually in order to avoid being punished by a wave.

Barrel: The hollow, tubular section of some waves.

Beach break: Waves that break near the shore.

Biomechanics: Refers to the joint and muscle positions used in a movement.

Blank: A large block of foam that is used to shape the core of most modern surfboards.

Blown out: When waves are flattened by strong wind.

Boneyard: The treacherous areas at surf spots; the term applies most often at shallow-water breaks.

Bottom turn: Turning the surfboard at the bottom of the wave face.

Break: Another name for a surf spot.

Chop: Ridges and bumps on the face of large waves.

Classic: Used to describe something traditional or timeless.

Cleanup set: A group of waves that are larger and may break farther out than what's been coming in; it usually catches people by surprise.

Close-out: A wave that breaks along the face all at once; it's not ideal for surfing.

Consistent: When sets of waves break regularly without a lot of downtime.

Crest: The top of a wave.

Cross stepping: Placing one foot in front of the other laterally to move forward or back on a longboard.

Curl: The area of the wave where the lip is falling and the wave is breaking.

Custom board: A board that is shaped to meet an individual's needs and style.

Cut back: A turn on the shoulder of the wave toward the breaking part of the wave.

Cutting off: Catching a wave in front of a surfer who is closer to the breaking part of the wave; aka dropping in or snaking; poor etiquette.

Deck: The top surface of the board, where a surfer stands.

Delaminate: When the fiberglass separates from the foam core of a surfboard.

Dig a rail: Falling as a result of putting too much body weight on one side of the surfboard.

Digger: A term used to describe a fall off a surfboard.

Ding: A puncture or dent in the board; it requires repair to avoid waterlog.

Drop: When a surfer takes off on a wave and is airborne at the beginning of a ride; it's most common in big and/or steep waves.

Dropping in: See "Cutting off"; poor etiquette.

Dry suit: A suit that doesn't let any water enter it; a waterproof suit.

Duck-dive: Submerging a board under water to get through an oncoming wave.

Face: The front side of the wave; what you see from the beach.

Flats: The less steep part of the wave away from the breaking part; also known as the shoulder.

Flex: Refers to how a snowboard or ski bends as it is weighted; this same concept is now being applied to some surfboards.

Floater: An advanced maneuver in which the surfer launches off the lip and rides the part of the wave that has broken.

Frontside: Surfing with your body facing the wave.

Funshape: A board that is usually between 7 and 9 feet long and has some of the characteristics of both a long- and shortboard; also called a hybrid.

Glassy: When waves are smooth as a result of very little or no wind action.

Glide: Used to describe how a longboard moves through water; how easy the board is to paddle and catch waves with.

Gnarly: A term used to describe big, heavy, or tough-to-ride waves.

Goofy foot: A stance in which your right foot is forward on the board.

Groms: Small kids who surf.

Gun: A board designed to be ridden in big waves; it's usually long and narrow.

Hammered: A term used to describe falling off a surfboard; also used to describe someone who is very drunk.

Hanging five: An advanced longboarding maneuver in which one foot (five toes) is placed on the very nose of the board.

Hanging ten: An advanced longboarding maneuver in which both feet (ten toes) are placed on the very nose of the board.

Haoles: A Hawaiian term for "nonlocals" or "whites."

Header: A term used to describe a fall off a surfboard.

Headstand: An advanced longboard surfing maneuver in which the rider is upside down.

He'enalu: An early Hawaiian term that means "wave sliding."

Helicopter: An advanced longboarding maneuver in which the board is spun around from the nose; also called a nose 360.

Hellmen, hellwomen: Surfers who ride big waves.

Hollow: A term used to describe a concave and steep wave face shape.

Hybrid: See "Funshape."

Impact zone: The area where the waves are breaking the hardest and most consistently.

Inside: The area between the impact zone and the shore.

Interference: When one surfer disrupts the ride of another who has the right-of-way during competition.

Interval training: A type of energy system workout involving periods of intensity followed by rest; it allows for more work to be performed at higher exercise intensities.

Kicking out: Turning out of a wave at the end of a ride.

Kook: An inexperienced or disrespectful surfer.

Leash: A cord used to tether the board to the surfer.

Lefts: Waves that break from the peak to the surfer's left; also called lefthanders.

Lines: Used to describe the swell as it approaches the shore.

Lineup: The area just outside of where the waves break; surfers wait here for waves.

Lip: The tip of the wave's peak that is breaking down the face.

Locals: Surfers who live near and surf a break on a regular basis.

Localism: When locals are hostile toward non-locals.

Longboard: A surfboard that's usually at least 9 feet long and has a round nose.

Lull: A period of time in which no waves or only very small waves are breaking.

Maxed out: When a surf spot is hit by waves that are too large to break without closing out.

Menehunes: A Hawaiian term for mythical leprechauns who fix or create problems; it's also used to refer to grom surfing categories.

Mush: When the waves are small and blown out.

Nose: The front section of a surfboard.

Nose 360: See "Helicopter."

Nose riding: Surfing on the front section of a longboard.

Offshore: A wind blowing from the shore toward the ocean; a light offshore is ideal in that it helps hold the wave faces up longer.

Off the lip: An advanced maneuver in which the board is turned at the lip of the wave.

Onshore: A wind blowing from the ocean toward the shore; a strong onshore will usually flatten waves and is not desirable.

Outline: The outer shape or silhouette of a surfboard.

Outside: The area between where the waves break and the open ocean.

Outside breaks: Areas where waves break that are farther from shore; when waves break at such spots, they tend to be larger than inside waves.

Overgunned: When a board is too big for the conditions.

Over the falls: When a surfer plunges down the wave face with the falling lip.

Pack: A large group of surfers in the lineup.

Peak: An area on the wave in relation to the shore where incoming waves are beginning to break; the ideal spot to catch waves.

Pearl: When the nose of the board submerges upon takeoff as a result of the surfer having too much weight forward.

Peeling: A wave whose lip crumbles gradually as it breaks.

Pit: The bottom of the wave; also known as the trough.

Pocket: The area just ahead of where the wave breaks; usually the steepest and most desirable place to surf.

Point break: When waves break on an area of land that juts out.

Popping up: Explosively moving from a prone position to standing when taking off on a wave.

Priority: Used to refer to a surfer who has wave precedence during competition.

Prone position: The facedown-lying position of a surfer paddling a surfboard.

Pumping: When medium- to large-sized waves are breaking consistently and with good shape.

Pumping the board: Forcing the board up and down while standing to generate speed on a wave.

Quiver: Refers to a surfer's board arsenal, with different sizes and shapes for varying conditions.

Rad: Short for "radical"; a slang term used to describe an impressive maneuver.

Rails: The side or turning edges of a surfboard.

Reef break: Waves that break over a reef, usually shallow; it's most common around islands.

Reentry: An advanced surfing maneuver performed off the lip of the breaking wave.

Reforms: Waves that have already broken and then build to break again.

Regular foot: A stance in which your left foot is forward on the board.

Rhino chaser: Another name for a "Gun"; a board used to attack large waves.

Rights: Waves that break from the peak to the surfer's right; also called righthanders.

Rip: A low spot in the shore where water flows back out toward the ocean after waves have broken.

Rocker: The upward curve at the nose or tail of a board.

Rogue wave: A wave that's much larger than the other waves in a swell.

Roller coaster: Surfing the whitewater that's created after a wave has broken.

Sand break: A surfing area where waves break over a sandbar.

Sea: Choppy waves in the open ocean created by a storm.

Section: A portion or area of a wave.

Set: A group of waves that approach the shore.

Setting up: Getting into an ideal position to perform a maneuver.

Shacked: Another term used to describe getting tubed.

Shaper: Someone who designs and makes surfboards.

Shortboard: A surfboard that's usually less than 7 feet long and has a pointed nose.

Shoulder: See "Flats."

Sideshore: Used to describe wind conditions in which the wind is blowing parallel to the breaking waves.

Slice 'n duck: A way to get a longboard through a broken wave, it involves putting the board on edge in order to submerge it under the whitewater.

Snaking: See "Cutting off"; poor etiquette.

Soup: See "Whitewater."

Spinout: Sliding sideways, usually as a result of the fin(s) losing contact with the wave face.

S stroke: A paddling technique in which the hands draw an S through the water.

Stall: Slowing a surfboard by pressuring the tail more than the nose.

Stick: A slang term for "surfboard."

Stoked: A term used by surfers to describe happiness.

Stringer: The middle strip of wood that runs the length of a surfboard; it's commonly made of balsa wood.

Sucky: Used to describe wave conditions that are "hollow" and breaking in shallow water.

Swell: Waves of energy that travel through the open ocean toward the shore.

Switch foot: A surfer who can surf both "goofy" and "regular" foot.

Switch-foot hop: An advanced surfing maneuver in which the rider jumps into the air, rotates 180 degrees, and lands facing the opposite direction.

Tail: The rear portion of a surfboard.

Takeoff: The act of catching and "Popping up" on a wave.

360: An advanced maneuver in which the board is spun around completely.

Thruster: A surfboard with three fins; also called a tri-fin.

Tide: Refers to the moon's effect on the depth of the water at different times of the day; tides can affect wave size and shape significantly.

Top-to-bottom: A type of wave that forms a tube; the lip is thrown out and all the way down the face.

Top turn: A maneuver in which the board is turned from high on the face toward the bottom.

Towing in: Using a motorized vehicle to sling a surfer into waves too large to catch by paddling.

Tri-fin: See "Thruster."

Trimming: Adjusting weight on a surfboard in order to keep it level and maximize speed.

Trough: See "Pit."

Tsunami: A monstrous wave that's formed by an underwater earthquake; these waves can be 100 feet tall and travel up to 600 miles per hour.

Tube: See "Barrel."

Turning radius: The distance a surfboard needs to make a direction change.

Turtle roll: The act of rolling a surfboard over to get through a breaking or broken wave.

Tweaked: A term used by surfers, skateboarders, and snowboarders to describe a variation on a maneuver; it's commonly used in aerial maneuvers.

Undergunned: When a board is too small for the conditions.

V: Refers to the convex shape of the bottom of a surfboard.

Wall: The smooth part of the wave face that hasn't broken.

Watermen, waterwomen: A term used to describe experienced and proficient ocean swimmers and surfers.

Wave height: The distance from the crest of a wave to the trough.

Wave length: The distance between two consecutive wave crests.

WaveRunner: A personal watercraft in which the rider is seated; it's used to tow in to large waves.

Wax: Rubbed onto the deck of a surfboard in order to provide traction for the surfer.

Wet suit: A neoprene suit that is worn to keep a surfer warm in cold water.

Whitewater: The frothy water that results after a wave breaks.

Wipeout: A fall while surfing.

Worked: A fall while surfing; it can also be used to describe a surfer who has been outsurfed by another.

Appendix B:

REFERENCES

Clark, Michael. *Integrated Training for the New Millennium.* Thousand Oaks, CA: National Academy of Sports Medicine, 2001.

Conway, John. *Adventure Sports Surfing.* Mechanicsburg, PA: Stackpole Books, 1988.

Hemmings, Fred. *The Soul of Surfing.* New York: Thunder's Mouth Press, 1997.

Werner, Doug. *Surfer's Start-Up: A Beginner's Guide to Surfing.* Chula Vista, CA: Tracks Publishing, 1993.

———. *Longboarder's Start-Up: A Guide to Longboard Surfing.* Chula Vista, CA: Tracks Publishing, 1996.

INDEX

About the Author

Raul Guisado has lived in California and played in the ocean all his life. He grew up surfing and skiing, splitting his time between Santa Cruz and Tahoe City. He has a B.A. in biological sciences from the University of California at Santa Barbara, is a certified strength and conditioning specialist, and is currently pursuing an M.A. in sports psychology. Raul has been coaching skiers and surfers since 1989 through his business Peak Athletic Coaching. From 1996 through 1999, he traveled the globe as a World Cup/Olympic coach for the U.S. Ski Team. He was a coach at the 1998 Olympic Winter Games in Nagano and at the 2002 Olympics in Salt Lake City, Utah. He hopes to one day coach surfing in the Olympics. For more information on coaching services, e-mail Raul at peakac@aol.com. Raul resides in Aptos, California.